TALI SHINE & LOHRALEE ASTOR

Feeding the Future

CLEAN EATING FOR CHILDREN & FAMILIES

teNeues

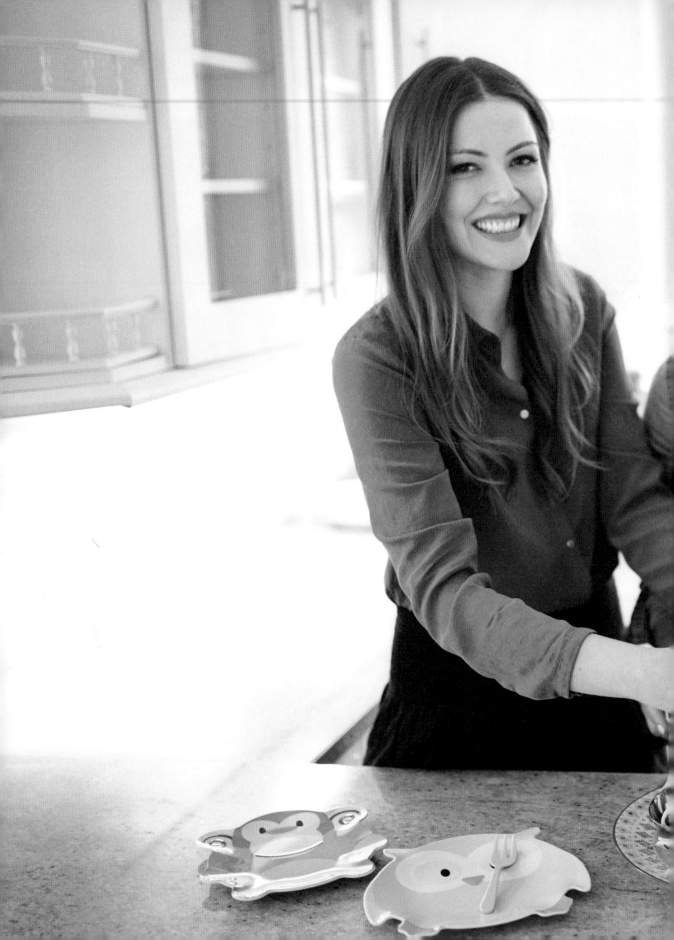

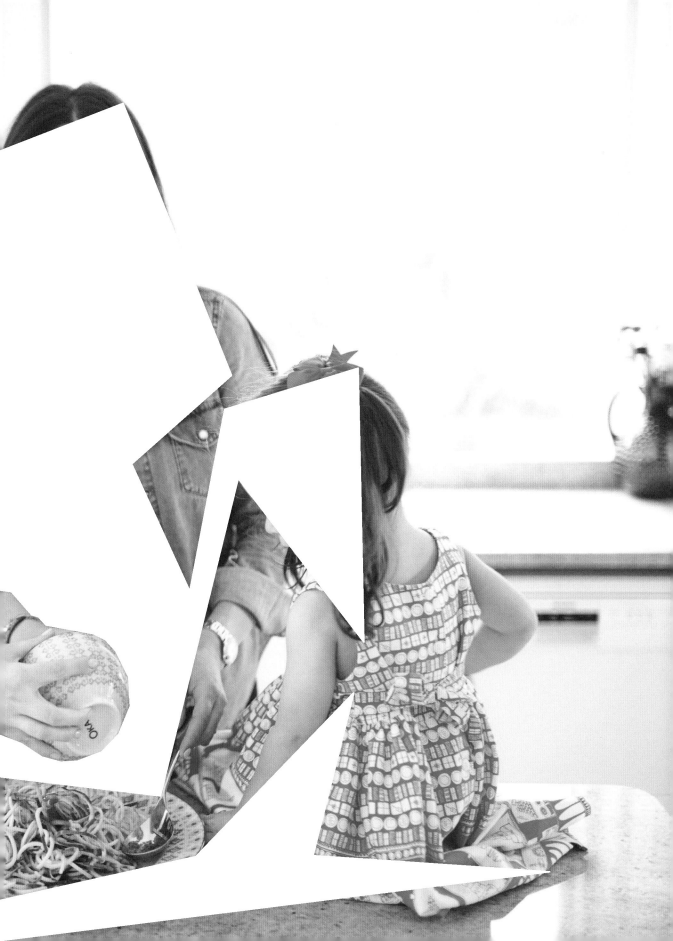

TABLE OF CONTENTS

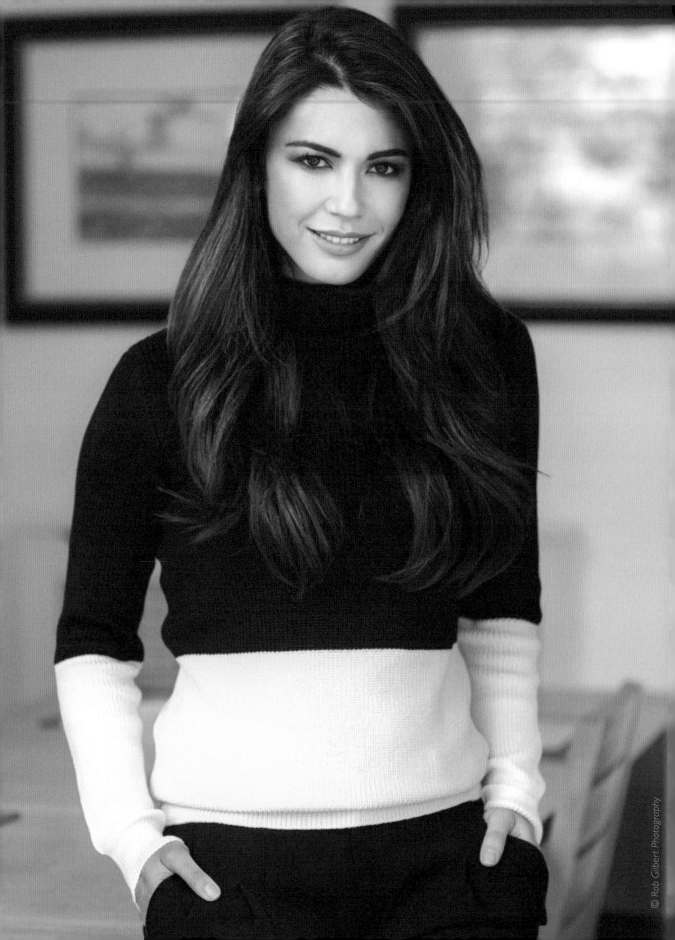

LOHRALEE ASTOR

Lohralee Astor's background as a nutritional therapist, as well as a wife and a mother to small children, has given her the perfect experience and tools to create delicious and healthy children's dishes. She has spent many hours practicing out of her Notting Hill clinic and advised various high-profile clients on their own diets, as well as those of their children.

Before she studied and landed her career in nutrition, Lohralee worked as a successful international model for v0 years, with prestigious clients including Guess, Diesel, and Lee Jeans. Her constant traveling and need to look her best inspired Lohralee to learn about the most effective ways to nourish and revitalise her body without compromising her health or well-being. It was then that her desire to find a healthier, balanced way of living was born. After studying and completing her diploma in nutrition from the College of Naturopathic Medicine in London, Lohralee extended her interest in nutrition and well-being into a career. She has contributed to UK-based children's e-magazine Ministylediary.com, where she created easy-to-make, healthy children's dishes and advised mothers on how to cook dishes that their children would actually eat.

Entertaining and cooking have always been some of Lohralee's great loves. She is often found in the kitchen of her West London home creating delicious, healthy dishes for her husband, Will, and her young children, Waldorf and Allegra. It has always been very important to Lohralee to instill healthy eating habits in her children to give them the foundation they need to grow and develop. She is constantly dreaming of new healthy recipes for her family, and the growing baby in her tummy that is due this spring.

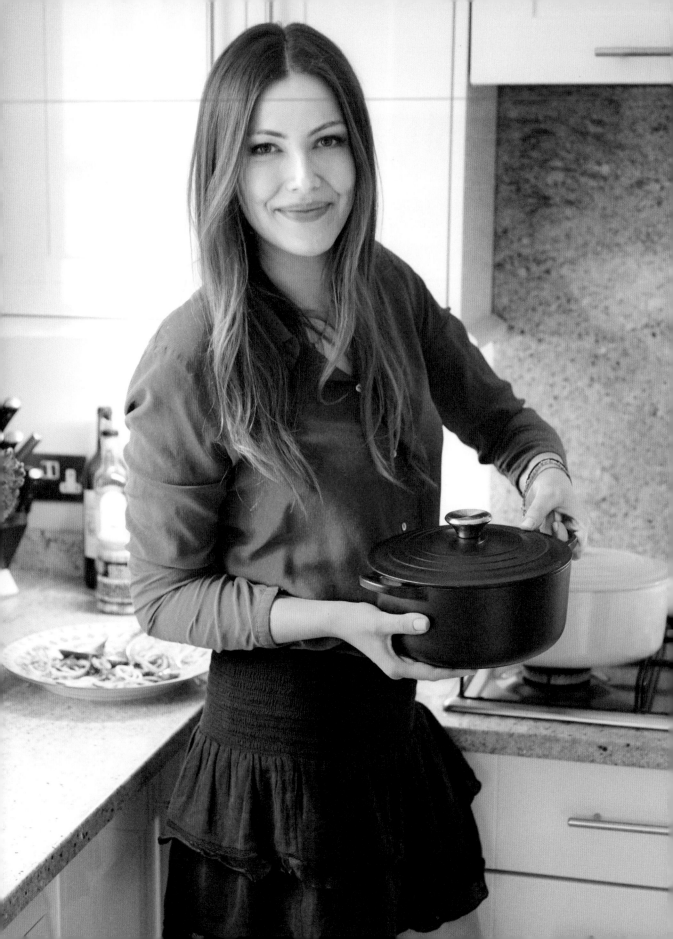

TALI SHINE

Author/presenter Tali Shine is a wellness, beauty, travel, health, and lifestyle expert who is based between Sydney and London.

Tali has commentated on-air and written for numerous magazines on health, beauty, nutrition, and new spa developments. As such, Tali has had the opportunity to interview and spend time with the world's leading lifestyle experts including scientists, fitness trainers, nutritionists, chefs, doctors, and therapists in order to learn about the newest and most exciting advancements in health, nutrition, and well-being.

Tali is a consultant with international spas and wellness centers, and was the head of health and wellness at London's prestigious South Kensington Club, helping to develop the spa, wellness program, and juice bar. She also worked with the clean eating franchise Counter Kitchen to help develop delicious on-the-go dishes and snacks for busy Londoners and their families.

In 2005, Tali created her own cosmetics line, Tali by Tali Shine, inspired by her favorite cities around the world. The line is available in Australia, the Philippines, Sweden, Canada, and the United Kingdom.

Tali's previous books include *The Glam Girl's Guide to Sydney Shopping*, *The Official Guide to NSW shopping*, and the clean eating recipe book *Good to Glow*.

Through her research and experience writing about clean eating, Tali saw how popular this way of life was becoming for adults. She also realized that children are the most vulnerable to additives and nasty toxins found in unhealthy, processed, and fast food. Seeing this issue, she began adjusting her recipes to cater to the tastes of her friend's young children to see if they would actually eat this type of food. She found that not only did they eat the dishes, they often asked for seconds!

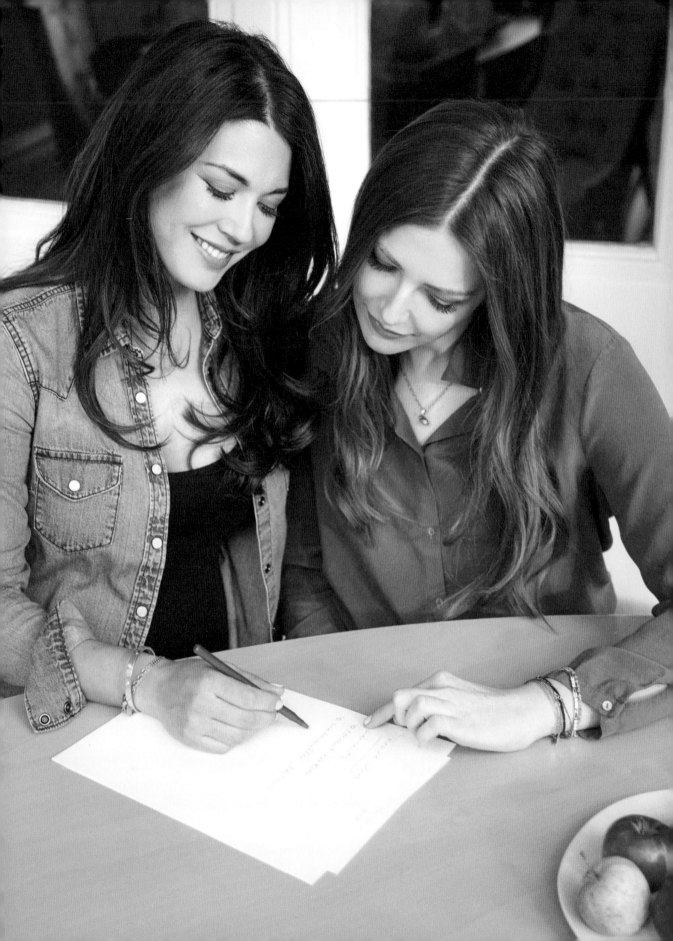

OUR STORY

The concept for *Feeding the Future* was created when Tali joined Lohralee and her family on holiday in the summer of 2015. Tali was working on her clean eating cookbook *Good to Glow* and going over many of the recipes with Lohralee, who was not only one of her closest friends, but also her trusted nutritionist.

The girls were discussing the nutritional content of the recipes and the importance of healthy eating when it occurred to them that while their friends were all clean eating converts, nutrition was even more vital for small children. The food that they eat affects their brain, the way they grow and function, and, most importantly, their future. It made no sense to the girls that so many parents gave their children processed food and sugar even though it can contribute to hyperactivity, poor concentration, behavior problems, and trouble sleeping.

Lohralee had always been vigilant about giving her children clean, nutrient-rich dishes. From the time her children ate their first solid food, she extensively planned creative meals for them every week in addition to advising her clients and friends on what to feed their children. Tali had also spent time coming up with fun, healthy dishes for a range of inter-national wellness venues, as well as for her godchildren, nieces, and nephews.

The girls decided to work together to create an ideal list of dishes for parents who want to ensure that their children have the most delicious, creative meals that are also easy to make. All of the dishes they created, developed, and tested are filled with nutrient-packed ingredients without ever compromising on taste. They're perfect for the fussiest of eaters, even with their mixture of special super-powers, vitamins, and vegetables smuggled into them.

Recipes were tested on Lohralee's children as well as run past Tali's little friends Coco, Rex, Raphaela, and Nathaniel. The girls altered the recipes to make sure that children of varying ages and tastes would enjoy the dishes. They cleverly developed recipes without refined sugar or harmful additives.

Lohralee also took into consideration that her son, Waldorf, has egg and dairy allergies. With this in mind, the girls thought up some recipes that would cater to Waldorf and other children with allergies similar to his. Tali and Lohralee know how important good food is and how significant it is to make sure that people feel included, especially during meal-time. This is the time for families and friends to meet and nurture a feeling of togetherness, which is especially important for children.

Keeping this in mind for families with other dietary needs, the girls have created plenty of allergy-conscious dishes easily categorized for you to find delicious alternatives. They have tagged pages to differentiate which recipes are dairy-free, egg-free, nut-free, and vegetarian, making it easy to plan menus. The girls hope you have as much fun preparing these recipes for your children as they did creating them!

OUR PRINCIPLES & SUPER INGREDIENTS

No Wheat Germ

Wheat germ can irritate the gut and may cause bacteria overgrowth and digestive issues. It may also affect the insulin levels in the body. Equilibrium in the body is essential, so correct insulin levels are necessary to maintain good health, body weight, and energy levels.

No Refined Sugar

Refined sugar is considered by many experts to be a highly addictive poison to the body. It's a pure, refined carbohydrate without any nutritional value. Sugar may cause irritability and poor concentration in children and contribute to hyperactivity and ADD symptoms. Instead of using refined sugar, we use healthier natural substitutes such as xylitol, maple syrup, rice malt syrup, coconut sugar, and dates.

No soy

Soy interferes with thyroxine (also known as T4) which is one of the main hormones that your thyroid produces. It is important to limit or avoid soy in your younger years as having a fully functional thyroid is crucial for healthy growth, metabolism, brain development, and bone maintenance.

Good Fats and Oils

We don't believe in avoiding fats. Instead, we replace bad fats with good fats which are necessary for the body and brain to function. We use coconut oil, olive oil, flaxseed oil, avocado oil, rapeseed oil, and avoid trans fats and saturated fats. We also believe in eating healthy omega-3 fats available in wild-caught salmon, oily fish, and seeds.

Almonds and Almond Milk

We use almonds and almond milk throughout our book as almonds are a rich source of protein, energy, and vitamins, such as vitamin E, calcium, zinc, selenium, and folate. Almonds are also a great source of manganese, potassium, iron, and magnesium. As almonds are free of gluten, they are a fantastic base for cooking for people with wheat and gluten intolerances and allergies.

Arrowroot Powder

Arrowroot powder, also known as arrowroot starch, is a white powdery ingredient derived from a tropical South American plant. The plant was given its name because it was once used to treat those injured with wounds from poison arrows. We use it as a natural thickener in recipes and to help sooth upset stomachs.

Avocados

Avocados are not only delicious, but they also have so many health benefits. We like to use them wherever we can to benefit from their high fiber and healthy fatty acids that have anti-inflammatory effects. Avocados are also incredibly high in potassium and contain protein, fiber, and vitamins K, C, E, B5, and B6. Avocado oil, like coconut oil, does not change considerable when it undergoes heat, making it good to cook with.

Bee Pollen

We like to consider bee pollen as the icing on our sugar-free cake. It is sweet and delicious on top of smoothies or baked goods, as well as mixed in with homemade nut butters. It is filled with many vitamins and can act as a natural antihistamine as it contains quercetin, which naturally works against allergies. Before use, it is important to test your child for bee pollen allergies and to discontinue use if your child demonstrates even the slightest allergy.

Blueberries

One of the most antioxidant rich food sources, blueberries are a delicious snack, and have a low glycemic index (therefore it doesn't spike our blood sugar levels). They act as a natural sweetener when added to smoothies, porridge, or muesli and may improve cognitive function including memory.

Chia Seeds

Chia seeds are a quick and easy-to-use source of protein and are filled with healthy fats, dietary fiber, minerals, vitamins, and antioxidants. They are completely vegan and don't go rancid as quickly as other seeds (they last up to two years when stored correctly). They also expand to make delicious puddings and jelly-like creations.

Coconut Oil

Coconut oil is a healthy fat that boasts antibacterial properties and can raise your good cholesterol. It's a great option for cooking, especially at high temperatures, as its nutritional benefits don't break down in high heat.

Flaxseeds

We try to sprinkle flaxseeds (also called linseeds) wherever we can. Throw them in cereal, cookies, and salads, or use them to make Super Seed Crackers for a hearty dose of alpha-linolenic acid, an essential fatty acid also known as ALA or omega-3. Flaxseeds are a great source of micro-nutrients, dietary fiber, manganese, magnesium, phosphorus, selenium, and vitamin B1. The other bonus is that flaxseeds are a lignin, which are fiber-like compounds and that have the same benefits as fiber and help to reduce bad cholesterol.

Goji Berries

Goji berries are little red berries that contain vitamin C, vitamin B2, vitamin A, iron, selenium, and antioxidants that can boost the immune system and may improve memory. The organic, dried version is a delicious snack and adds natural sweetness when included in dishes.

Himalayan Pink Salt

Himalayan pink salt is believed to be the purest salt on earth. This salt is hand-mined from the Himalayan mountains that stretch across Asia. This type of salt is rich in iodine and also contains small amounts of potassium, calcium, iron, and magnesium while boasting slightly lower levels of sodium than table salt.

Lemons

We love using lemons because they are packed with folate and contain high amounts of vitamin C which strengthens the immune system, helping to prevent colds and the flu. It also acts as a great replacement for salt.

Maple Syrup

The sweet fluid is sap that has been drilled out of maple trees, then boiled until most of its water evaporates. What's left is a thick syrup that gets filtered to remove impurities. This sweetener contains vitamins and minerals including B2, calcium, potassium, as well as antioxidants.

Millet

Millet is a gluten-free grain that can be enjoyed as a traditional cereal, to make porridge, or to cook bread. Millet is high in B vitamins, which boost your energy and metabolism while supporting your nervous system regulation. Millet also contains many important minerals such as magnesium, potassium, zinc, copper, manganese, and phosphorus, which is important for bone support.

Oats (Whole and Gluten-Free)

Oats are a fantastic source of fiber, including a special fiber known as beta-glucan that helps remove cholesterol from the digestive system and stabilize blood sugar levels. Oats will give your children a sustained release of energy thanks to their complex carbohydrates. We choose either whole oats (these do contain gluten) or gluten-free oats if your children have gluten allergies.

Raw or Manuka Honey

Raw honey contains bee pollen, B vitamins, anti-inflammatory properties, minerals, and enzymes. Manuka honey is great to have when you're not feeling well as it is known for its anti-bacterial properties. The honey must be rated 10 UMF or be active Manuka honey to have its anti-bacterial effect. Raw honey is excellent for baking, but because it is raw (unprocessed), it is not recommended for children under two.

Rice Malt Syrup

Rice malt syrup is a great natural sweetener that is made from fermented, cooked rice and is basically glucose. Glucose is found in starchy food and it is not considered harmful like fructose.

Sea Salt

Sea salt is also high in iodine. Sea salt undergoes only a little processing unlike normal table salt. The clearer the sea salt, the more pure it is.

Xylitol

Xylitol is a natural sweetener extracted from birch wood. It has forty percent less calories than sugar. It's suitable for people with diabetes thanks to its low glycemic index which means that it doesn't cause a spike in insulin levels. It is also renowned for helping to prevent tooth decay and repair damage to tooth enamel.

ALLGERY INFORMATION

Key to recipe icons:

 Dairy-free

 Egg-free

 Gluten-free

 Peanut-free

 Shellfish-free

V Vegan

DRINKS

*Not only are our juices, smoothies, and nut milks
easy to make and filled with calcium, vitamins,
and minerals, they are also perfect for kids. Sometimes
getting your kids to eat healthy foods is not that simple.
Creamy smoothies and naturally sweetened nut milks
are delicious and nutritious. What's more, green juices
and smoothies are perfect ways to hide veggies that
your kids may not eat on their own.*

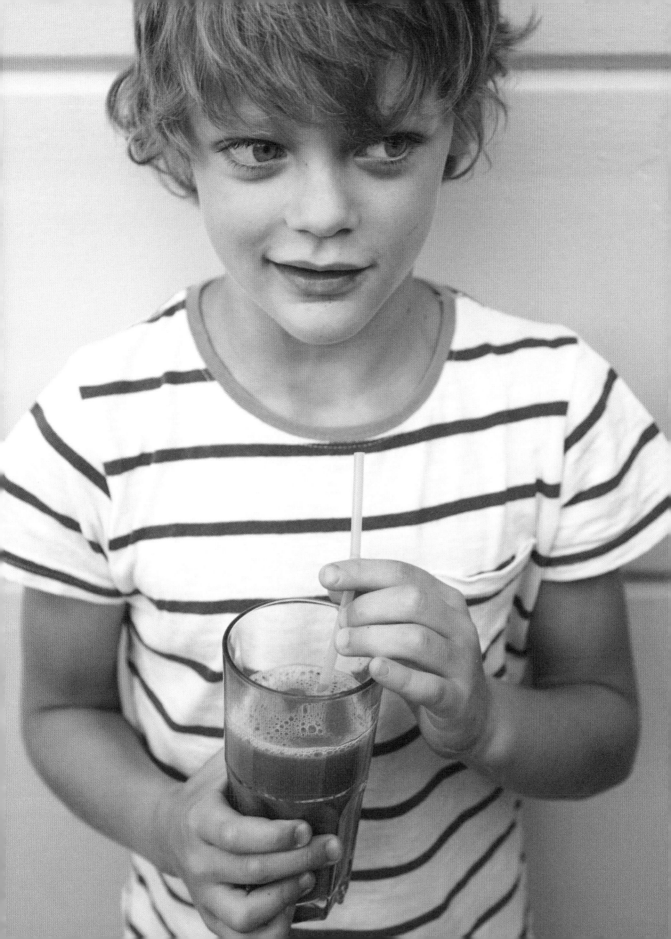

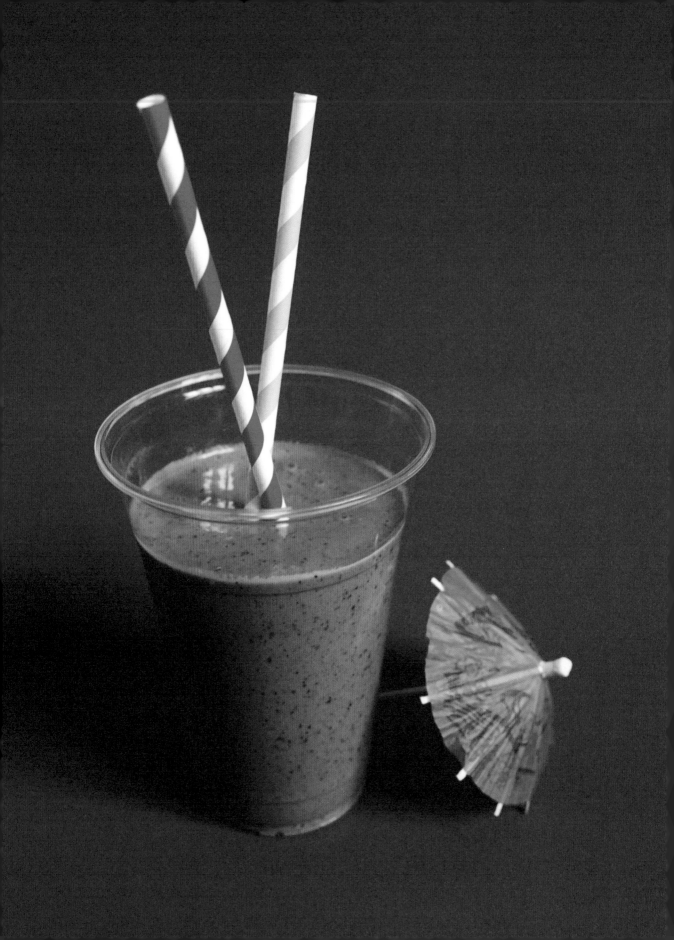

FROZEN SMOOTHIE

Elsa and Anna from the movie, Frozen, would be delighted with this smoothie. It is packed with protein, which will help you maintain energy throughout the day, as well as potassium, antioxidants, and magnesium. It is perfect for a long day at school or a nature trek.

INGREDIENTS

- 1 frozen banana
- ½ cup / 65 g frozen blueberries
- 480 ml / 2 cups Almond Milk (unsweetened) (see recipe page 20)
- 1 tbsp ground flaxseed
- 1 tbsp bee pollen
- 1 tbsp FTF Almond Butter (see recipe page 161)
- 1 oz / 28 g raw cacao powder
- Ice cubes

PREPARATION

PUT all ingredients in a high-speed blender and blend until smooth.

ADD a handful of ice cubes.

YOGI BERRY SMOOTHIE

Sweet and delicious, this smoothie is an excellent morning energy kick or afternoon snack. Packed with antioxidants, protein, and vitamin C, it will ensure that your kids are smarter than the average bear!

INGREDIENTS

- 2 cups / 260 g mixed berries (blueberries, strawberries, blackberries)
- 1 ripe pear
- 1 cup / 240 ml Almond Milk (see recipe page 20)
- ¼ cup / 30 g goji berries
- 1 tsp chia seeds

PREPARATION

WASH berries and pear thoroughly.

ADD all the ingredients to a blender and mix until smooth.

WHAT'S UP DOC JUICE

The vitamin C and antioxidants in this juice will give your kids more energy than Bugs Bunny!

INGREDIENTS

- 3 carrots
- ⅜ in / 1 cm fresh ginger
- ⅜ in / 1 cm fresh turmeric
- 1 peeled orange

PREPARATION

WASH all the ingredients and put through a juicer.

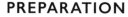

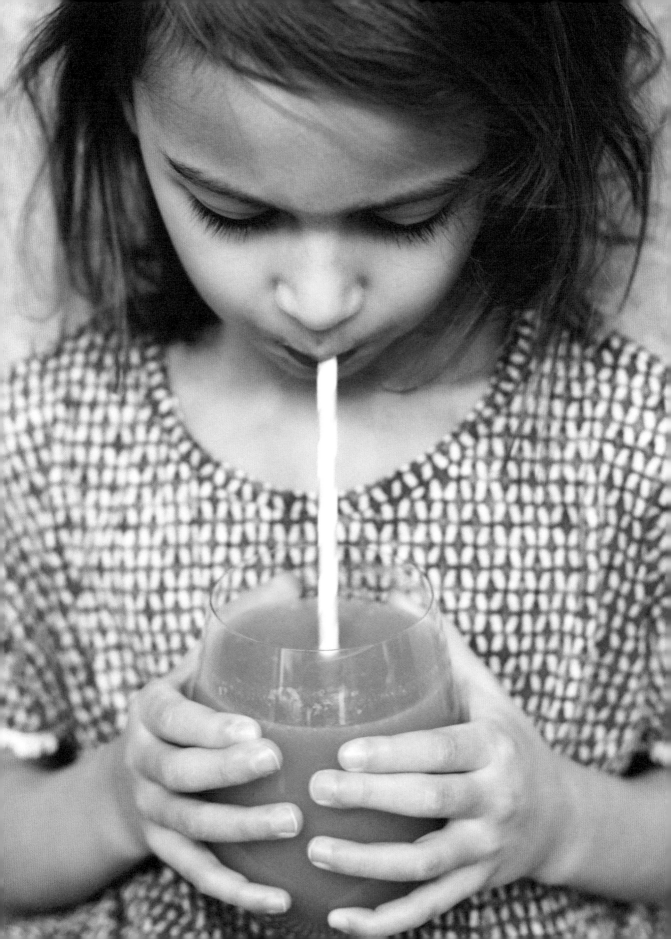

ALMOND MILK

Filled with selenium, protein, and zinc, this easy-to-make almond milk is delicious on its own, or flavored with something extra like berries or raw cacao.

INGREDIENTS

- 1 ½ cups / 215 g almonds
- 3 cups / 720 ml filtered water
- 1 pinch Himalayan pink salt
- 1 tbsp maple syrup
- ¼ vanilla bean (optional)
- 2 dates (optional)
- Dash of cinnamon (optional)

PREPARATION

PLACE the almonds in a bowl and cover with water.

COVER the bowl and leave overnight (8 to 12 hours).

In the morning, DRAIN and RINSE the almonds with water.

PLACE the almonds in a blender with 1 cup / 240 ml of water and blend.

ADD 2 more cups / 480 ml of water, salt, maple syrup, vanilla bean (optional), and dates (optional).

BLEND on high until the nuts are smooth (approximately 2 minutes), then let the mixture sit for 5 minutes.

STRAIN the mixture through a nut milk bag (available from health food shops as well as online). KEEP the almond meal to use as a raw cookie mixture.

PLACE milk in a glass jar and store in the fridge for up to five days.

OAT MILK

Easy to make and filled with fiber, this homemade milk can be used for cooking, in cereals, or in smoothies.

INGREDIENTS

- 1 ½ cups / 235 g oats
- 3 cups / 720 ml filtered water
- 1 pinch Himalayan pink salt
- 1 tbsp maple syrup
- ¼ vanilla bean (optional)

PREPARATION

PLACE the oats in a bowl and cover with water.

COVER the bowl and leave overnight (8 to 12 hours).

In the morning, DRAIN and RINSE the oats with water.

PLACE the oats in a blender with 1 cup / 240 ml of water and blend.

ADD 2 more cups / 480 ml of water, salt, maple syrup, and vanilla bean (optional).

BLEND on high until the oats are smooth (approximately 30 seconds), then let the mixture sit for 5 minutes.

STRAIN the mixture through a nut milk bag (available from health food shops as well as online).

PLACE milk in a glass jar and store in the fridge for up to five days.

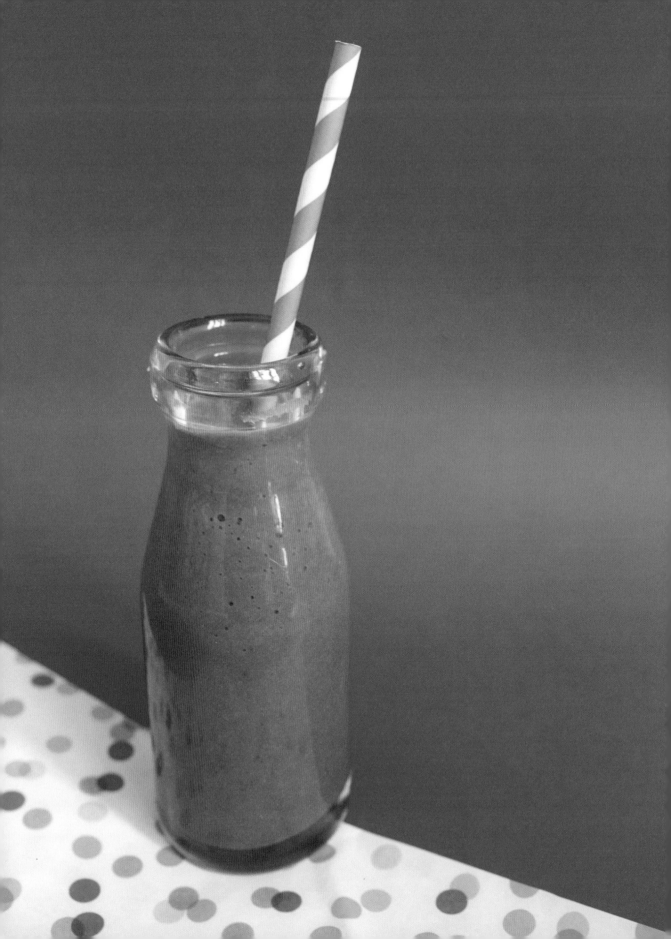

SUPER HERO JUICE

A great way to get your children to take in their greens is through juicing. This juice is high in antioxidants and vitamin K, which is important for bone development. If only they knew how good juice is for them!

INGREDIENTS

- 2 celery sticks
- 1 handful of spinach
- 1 apple
- 1 cup / 180 g pomegranate seeds

PREPARATION

WASH celery, spinach, and apple thoroughly.

POP all the ingredients into a juicer and you're good to go! Enjoy!

HUG IN A MUG HOT COCOA

This hot chocolate will bring a smile to kids of all ages. Coconut oil is filled with healthy good fats and also creates a creamy, frothy texture. Cinnamon has many health benefits and complements the maple syrup, raw honey, or rice malt syrup, without the need for refined sugar.

INGREDIENTS

- 2 cups / 480 ml Almond Milk (see recipe page 20)
- 1 tbsp raw cacao
- 1 tbsp maple syrup, raw honey, or rice malt syrup
- 1 tbsp coconut oil
- ½ tsp cinnamon

PREPARATION

HEAT the almond milk on the stovetop to just under boiling point.

ADD the remaining ingredients and whisk.

HEAT on medium for another 2 minutes and serve.

BERRY TEA

Sweet and delicious, this tea tastes like a treat and is filled with vitamin C and antioxidants!

INGREDIENTS

- 1 handful seasonal berries (finely chopped) (we love strawberries, blueberries, and raspberries)
- Small amount of Manuka honey to taste
- Filtered water

PREPARATION

WASH and rinse the chopped berries.

PLACE berries in a teapot.

MELT a small amount of Manuka honey into filtered water.

POUR the honey and boiling water into the teapot and let berries infuse the water for a couple of minutes. The water may change to a reddish color.

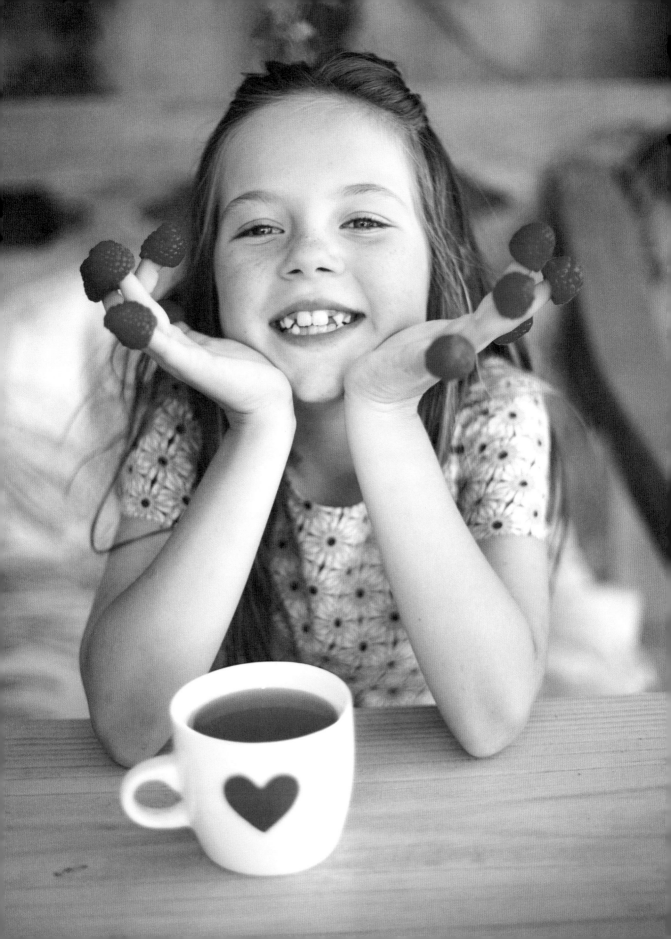

GINGER KISS TEA

Like a warm kiss on a winter's day, this tea is soothing, plus it's filled with vitamin C as well as anti-inflammatory properties!

INGREDIENTS

- 2 medium pieces of ginger
- Filtered water
- Manuka honey to taste

PREPARATION

REMOVE the skin from the ginger.

GRATE or SLICE the ginger into medium sized pieces.

PLACE ginger in a teapot and add boiled, filtered water.

LEAVE the ginger and add Manuka honey to taste.

This drink can also be served cold as a juice.

CINNAMON TEA

Kiddies love having a cup of cinnamon tea first thing in the morning. Try bringing them a cup of tea with a Ginger Snap Cookie (see recipe page 54) on the weekend or school holidays!

INGREDIENTS

- 4 ¼ cups / 1 l filtered water
- 2 cinnamon sticks (crushed)
- 1 tsp Manuka honey

PREPARATION

CRUSH the cinnamon sticks with a mortar and pestle, and put into a teapot (we use a teapot with an internal strainer).

ADD boiling water and 1 teaspoon of Manuka honey.

LET tea sit for 5 minutes before serving.

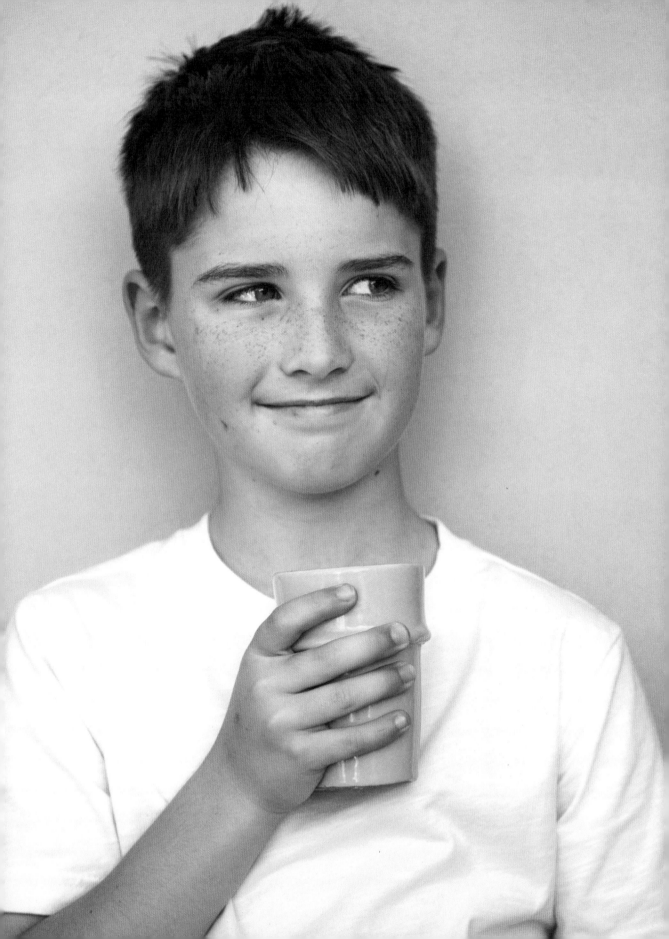

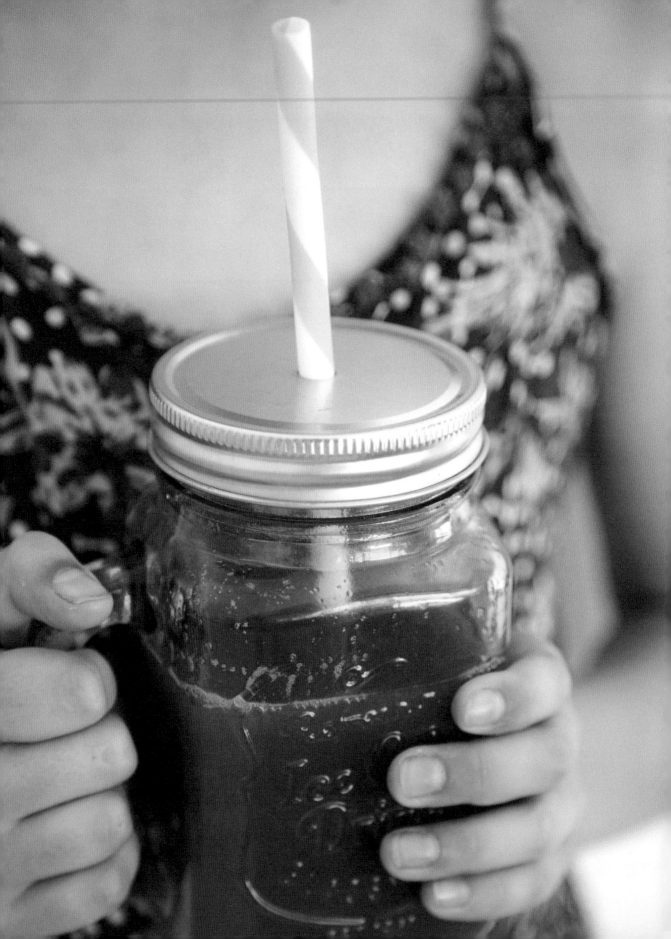

MERMAID SMOOTHIE

This under the sea delight is filled with iron, protein, potassium, and healthy fats. It is rich and creamy while nourishing the body. Enjoy as a snack or a special treat.

INGREDIENTS

- 1 small fistful of kale
- 1 small fistful of baby spinach
- ¼ of an avocado
- ¼ of a mango
- ½ medium banana
- 1 cup / 240 ml coconut water
- 5 dates (chopped)

PREPARATION

WASH kale and spinach thoroughly.

ADD all the ingredients to a blender and mix until smooth.

BREAKFAST

Breakfast is the most important meal of the day, especially for children. You are literally breaking a fast! After not eating for 8 to 12 hours during the night, your body and brain need fuel. Without a nutritious breakfast, children can be restless, grumpy, find it hard to focus, and tire easily.

As breakfast is such a crucial meal, it is particularly important to feed your children whole grains, fiber, calcium, and other wholesome nutrients we've included in our recipes. This can increase their energy and may help their physical activities and concentration. We hope this will help them do better in school, and of course eat healthier throughout the day.

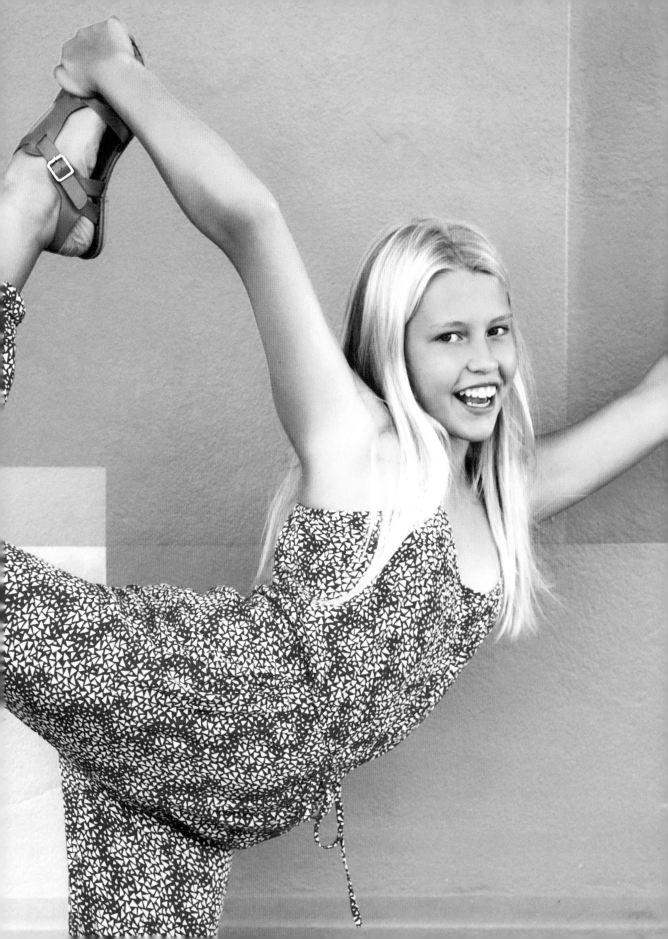

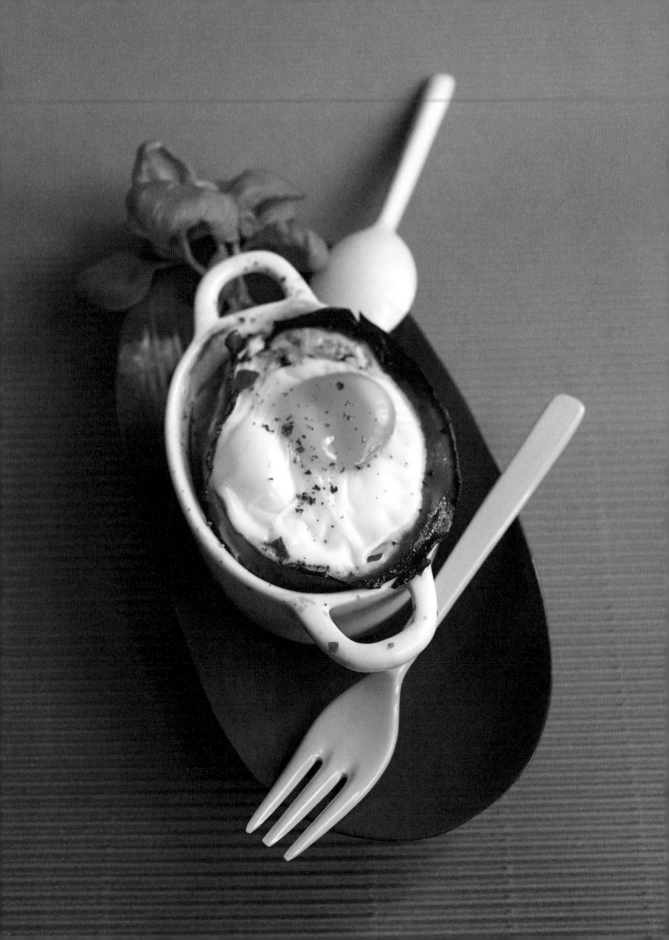

BAKED EGGS

This dish is easy peasy. Eggs are a simple way to get all the nutrients your growing mini needs to be healthy and strong. Eggs provide a complete range of amino acids and complete protein. This means a dream child.

INGREDIENTS

- 1 tbsp of tomato puree
- 3 cherry tomatoes
- 1 basil leaf
- 1 slice of ham (optional)
- 1 egg

PREPARATION

PREHEAT oven to 390°F / 200°C.

MIX the tomatoes, tomato puree, and basil in a blender.

ADD mixture from the blender to the dishes with the ham (optional).

CRACK the egg in your small baking dish.

BAKE for 12 to 15 minutes.

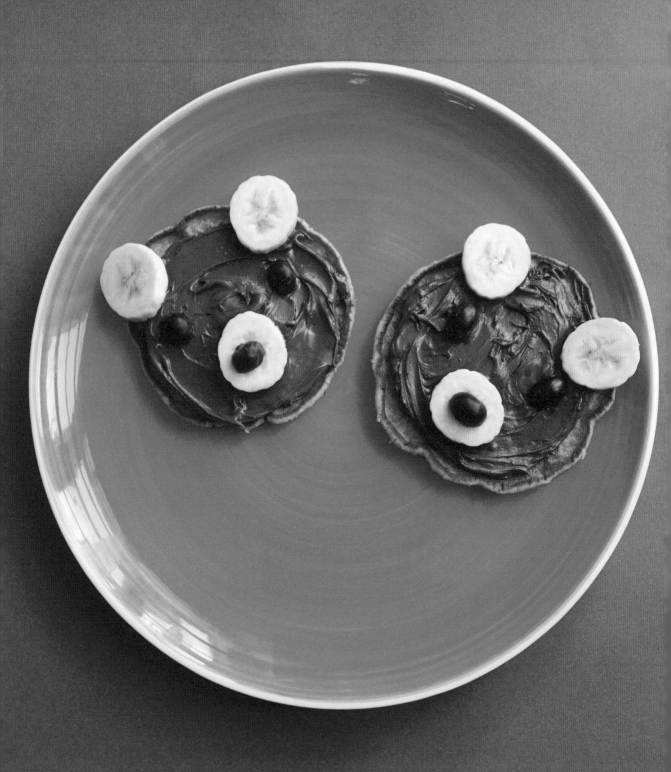

BANANA OAT PANCAKES
& UN-NUTELLA

This yummy scrummy dish will have your kids fighting over the last bite. The oats in these pancakes are filled with fiber and the bananas are rich in potassium. The cottage cheese is loaded with protein and calcium making this a delicious and perfectly balanced first meal of the day. Better yet, they are so easy to make!

INGREDIENTS

- Coconut oil for cooking
- 1 ¼ cup / 200 g gluten-free rolled oats (you can also use whole oats, but keep in mind these contain gluten)
- 4 eggs
- 1 scant cup / 100 g cottage cheese
- Un-Nutella (see recipe page 36), cinnamon, banana, or berries for garnish

PREPARATION

BLEND the ingredients in a food processor.

HEAT a nonstick pan at medium heat, then add coconut oil to the pan.

POUR ingredient mixture into the heated pan by the ¼ cup / 60 ml.

COOK until you see little bubbles that stay popped (roughly 2 to 3 minutes per side).

SERVE with Un-Nutella, a sprinkle of cinnamon, banana slices, or fresh berries.

BANANA OAT PANCAKES
& UN-NUTELLA

INGREDIENTS

- 1 cup / 150 g hazelnuts
- ⅓ cup / 75 ml coconut milk (full cream)
- ¼ cup / 80 ml maple syrup
- 1 tsp vanilla bean paste
- 2 tbsp raw cacao powder

PREPARATION

PREHEAT oven to 350°F / 180°C.

PLACE hazelnuts on a lined baking tray and roast for approximately 10 to 12 minutes. Be careful not to burn them!

LET the hazelnuts cool completely, then rub away their skins with a paper towel.

In a food processor, BLEND hazelnuts until they become a nut butter.

ADD remaining ingredients to the food processor and blend until smooth.

VEGAN PANCAKES

Easy-to-make and delicious, these pancakes are perfect for vegans and those with egg or dairy allergies. Serve alone or get creative with toppings like blueberries and maple syrup for some sweetness.

INGREDIENTS

- 1 ¼ cup / 150 g gluten-free, self-rising flour
- ½ tsp salt
- 1 ¼ cup / 300 ml Oat Milk (see recipe page 21)
- 1 tsp olive oil
- Coconut oil for cooking

PREPARATION

SIFT the flour and salt into a large bowl.

WHISK the oat milk and oil together in a small bowl.

MAKE a hole in the center of the dry ingredients, and then pour in the oat milk and olive oil.

BLEND the mixture together (batter will be lumpy).

HEAT a lightly oiled pan over medium-high heat.

DROP the batter into the pan with a large spoon and cook until bubbles form and the edges are dry.

FLIP and COOK until browned on the other side.

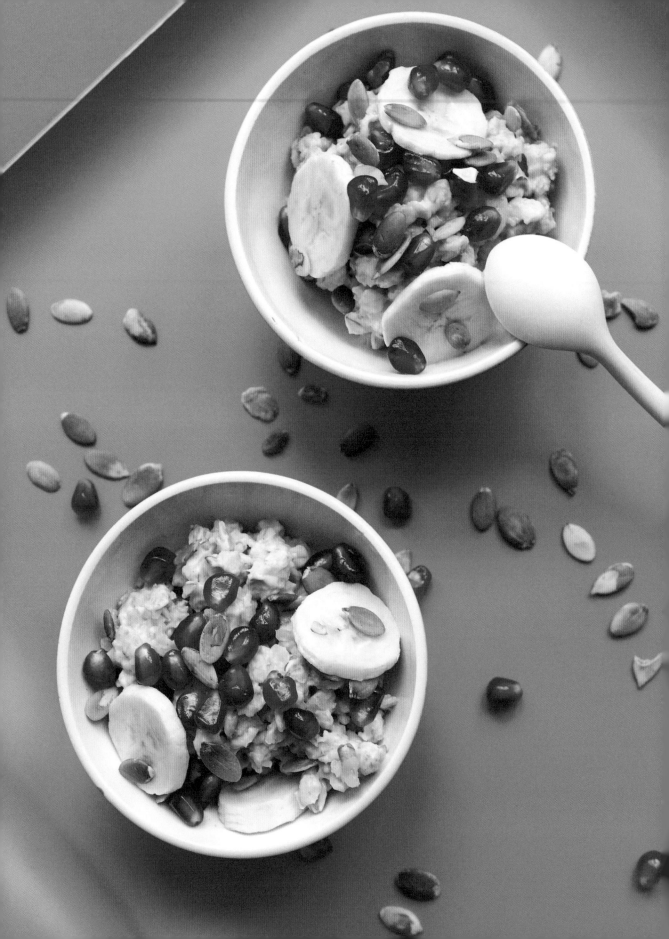

PORRIDGE

A healthy source of fiber and a great way to start the day, porridge is filling, immune boosting, and delicious.

INGREDIENTS

- 1 cup / 90 g gluten-free oats, whole rolled oats (if you don't have a problem with gluten), or a substitute such as rice or quinoa flakes
- 2 cups / 500 ml filtered water
- 1 pinch sea salt
- ½ cup / 125 ml Almond Milk (see recipe page 20) or filtered water
- Choice of Manuka honey, maple syrup, blueberries, banana, cinnamon, or goji berries for garnish

PREPARATION

SOAK oats overnight with 1 cup / 240 ml of water (soaking optional).

COMBINE soaked oats and 1 cup / 240 ml of water, or dry oats and 2 cups / 480 ml of water in a small saucepan.

ADD a pinch of sea salt and stir continuously over medium heat until mixture boils.

SIMMER, continuously stirring, for 3 to 5 minutes or until thick.

ADD almond milk or water and stir until heated through.

DIVIDE porridge among bowls and top with an assortment of recommended garnish ingredients.

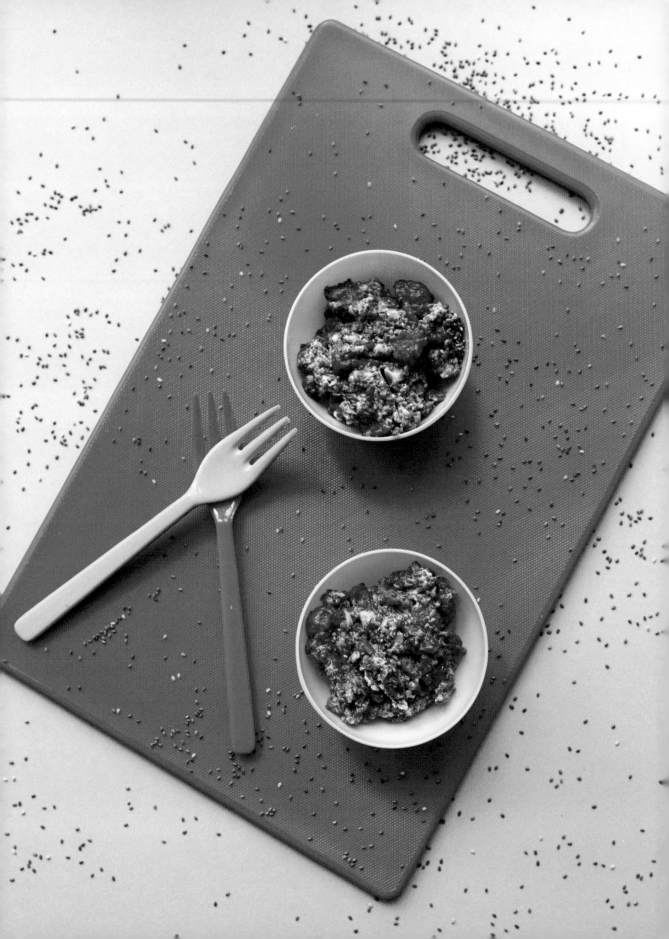

CHIA BREAKFAST POT

This pot is high in antioxidants, rich in fiber, vitamins C, E, B1, B3, B5, and B6 and minerals including iron, selenium, sodium, calcium, magnesium, and phosphorous. It is also delicious and looks amazing when served.

INGREDIENTS

- ¼ cup / 40 g chia seeds
- 1 cup / 75 g coconut cream
- ½ cup / 65 g blueberries
- 1 tsp vanilla extract
- 2 tsp Manuka honey
- 1 tbsp hazelnuts (crushed)
- 1 tbsp almond shavings
- ¼ cup / 30 g mixed raspberries and blueberries
- 2 tbsp coconut shavings

PREPARATION

COMBINE chia seeds, coconut cream, blueberries, vanilla extract, and honey in a bowl.

MIX well, cover, and refrigerate overnight or for a few hours before serving.

SCATTER crushed hazelnuts and almond slices, top with some extra blueberries, raspberries, and coconut shavings to serve.

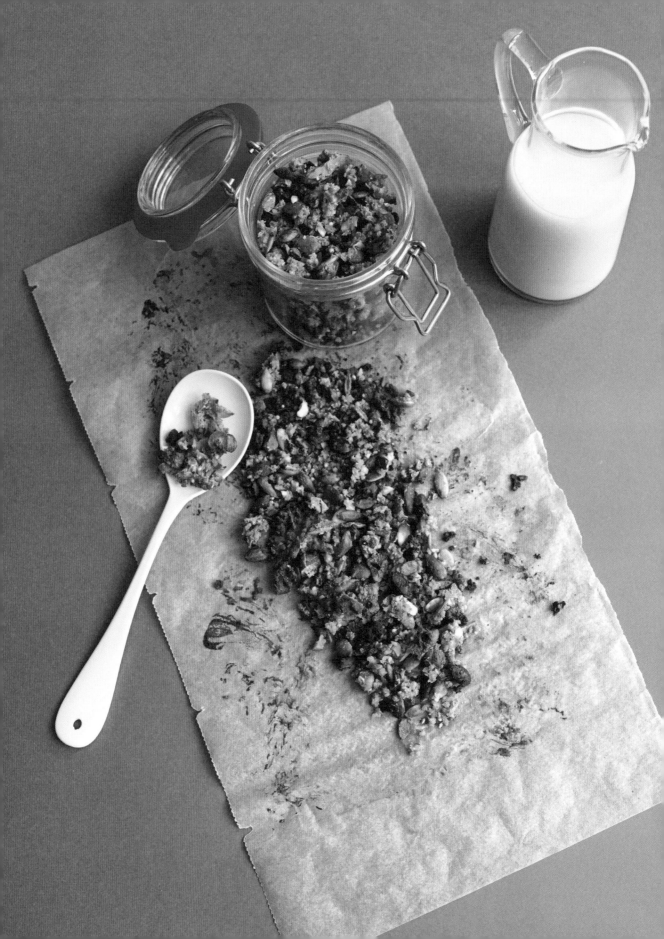

MILLET GRANOLA

Millet is a super grain! It's nutrient-dense with copper (which helps build strong tissues), manganese, phosphorus, and magnesium. This grain also contains lignin, which is an antioxidant. We should actually call this "Super Granola" because that is exactly what it is!

INGREDIENTS

- 2 cups / 340 g sprouted millet
- ½ cup / 50 g walnuts (chopped)
- ½ cup / 50 g pecans (chopped)
- ¼ cup / 30 g pumpkin seeds
- 3 tsp cinnamon
- 1 pinch of ground cardamom
- ¼ tsp nutmeg
- 4 tbsp maple syrup
- 3 tbsp tahini
- 1 tsp vanilla extract

PREPARATION

PREHEAT the oven to 350°F / 180°C.

COMBINE all wet ingredients in a bowl.

POUR the wet ingredients into a large mixing bowl with the millet, cinnamon, nutmeg, and cardamom until granola has formed.

SPREAD the granola evenly on a baking tray.

BAKE for 15 minutes, then stir and add the nuts.

BAKE for another 10 minutes, keeping a close eye on the texture and cooking status.

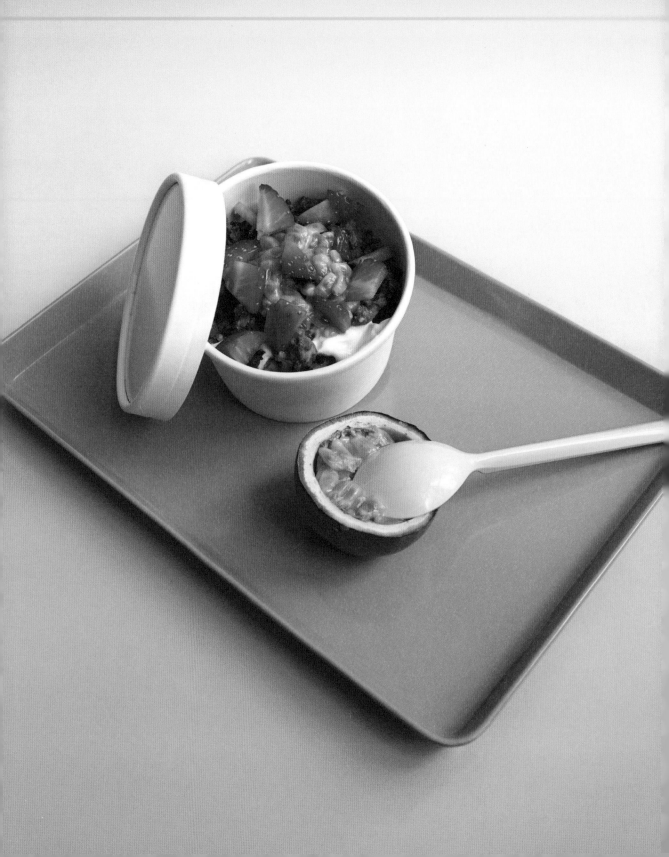

MILLET BREAKFAST POT

This breakfast recipe is so popular that if you turn away for a second, it will be gone! Full of color and antioxidants, this yummy scrummy dish is an easy throw together breakie when you are in a rush. You may also choose to use it as a dessert.

INGREDIENTS

(Serves 2)

- 🍎 1 cup / 180 g pomegranate seeds
- 🍎 1 cup / 245 g coconut yogurt
- 🍎 2 passion fruits (deseeded)
- 🍎 1 cup / 120 g millet granola (see recipe page 42)

PREPARATION

PLACE ½ cup / 90 g of pomegranate seeds into each bowl.

ADD ½ cup / 120 g of coconut yogurt, 1 passion fruit, and ½ cup / 60 g of millet granola.

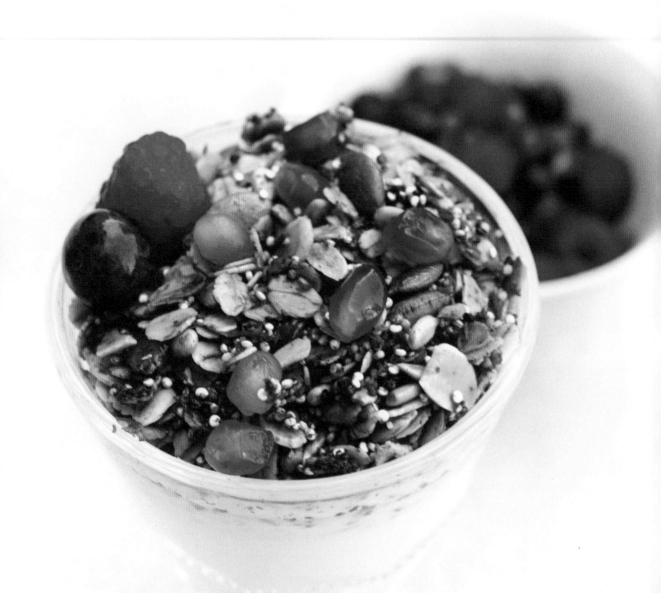

GRANOLA

This is a traditional granola without all of the refined sugar. A bit of cinnamon in the mix helps to maintain blood sugar levels and the oats are a great source of fiber, magnesium, and chromium. This granola is so popular that we actually need to hide it from some people, and let's just say it's not the children!

INGREDIENTS

- ¼ cup / 60 ml agave nectar
- ⅓ cup / 100 ml maple syrup
- 4 tbsp rapeseed oil
- ½ tsp sea salt
- 1 tsp cinnamon
- 3 tbsp water
- 3 ¼ cups / 300 g gluten-free oats, whole rolled oats (if you don't have a problem with gluten), or a substitute such as rice or quinoa flakes
- ½ cup / 60 g Brazil nuts (chopped)
- ½ cup / 60 g pecans (chopped)
- ⅓ cup / 80 g walnuts (chopped)
- ¼ cup / 30 g dried cranberries
- ¼ cup / 30 g dried blueberries

PREPARATION

PREHEAT the oven to 285°F / 140°C.

LINE a baking tray with baking parchment and set aside.

MIX together the salt, cinnamon, water, rapeseed oil, agave nectar, and maple syrup into a pan and gently cook until you see tiny little bubbles (do not boil).

ADD the oats and mixture from the pan in a large mixing bowl.

MIX until the all the oats are coated with the sauce from the pan.

POUR the mixture onto your baking sheet and cook for 30 minutes, mixing the granola every 10 minutes.

After 30 minutes, ADD the nuts so they become golden and crispy (this should take about 10 minutes).

Once the granola is cooked, REMOVE it from the oven and mix in the dried berries.

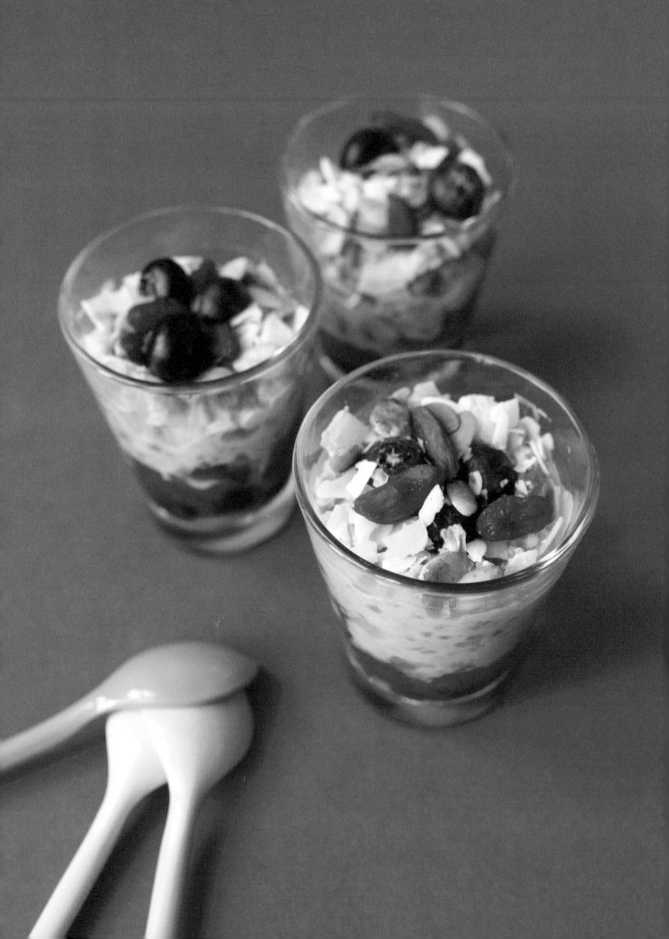

SUMMER BIRCHER MUESLI

This is the perfect dish for a summer day. It looks like pure sunshine and tastes delicious, while still being filled with fiber, protein, omegas, and vitamin C!

INGREDIENTS

- 2 cups / 180 g gluten-free oats
- 2 tbsp white chia seeds
- 2 cups / 480 ml unfiltered apple juice
- 3 tbsp coconut milk
- 2 tbsp almonds (sliced)
- 2 tbsp coconut (shredded)
- 2 tbsp pumpkin seeds
- 1 ½ cups / 350 g coconut yogurt
- 1 tbsp maple syrup
- 2 Granny Smith apples (grated)
- 1 cup / 180 g pomegranate seeds
- 1 cup / 130 g blueberries
- Cinnamon to taste

PREPARATION

ADD oats, apple juice, coconut milk, and chia seeds to a bowl and gently stir to combine.

PLACE the bowl in the refrigerator and soak overnight.

SET aside a small amount of the coconut, almonds, pumpkin seeds, pomegranate, and blueberries for garnish.

In the morning, MIX in the grated apples, coconut yogurt, maple syrup, shredded coconut, almonds, pumpkin seeds, blueberries, pomegranate seeds, and cinnamon.

REFRIGERATE for an hour.

GARNISH with reserved nuts, seeds, and fruits as desired.

SWEET SNACKS

Sweet snacks can be given as a special treat, and
we all love treats! The great news is that even
sweet snacks can be healthy and nutritious.
FTF snacks are made with love and packed full of
antioxidants. Our sweet treats are free of refined sugar
and all of these super snacks have a nutritious punch
to them.

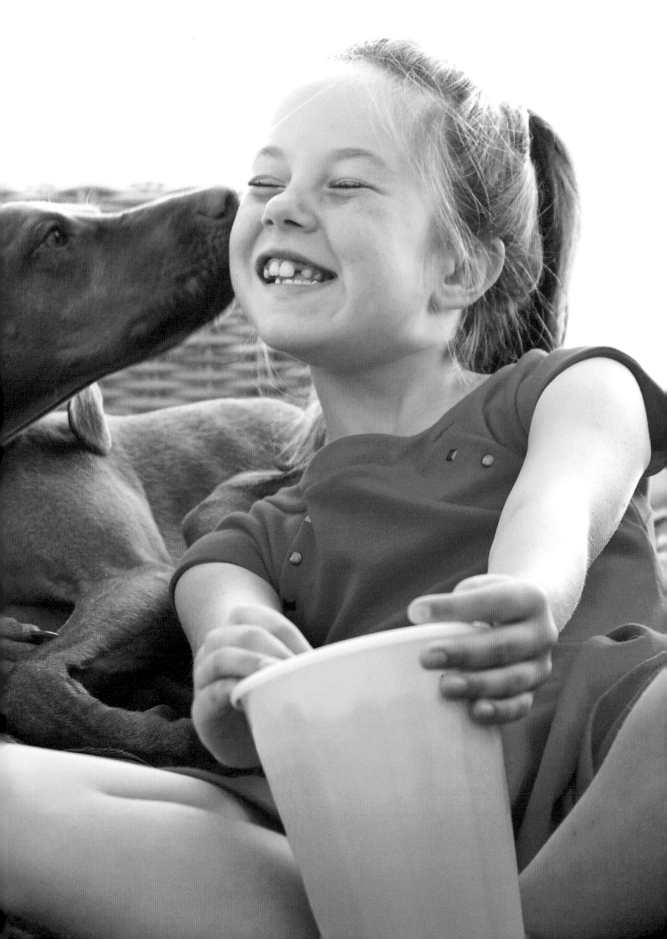

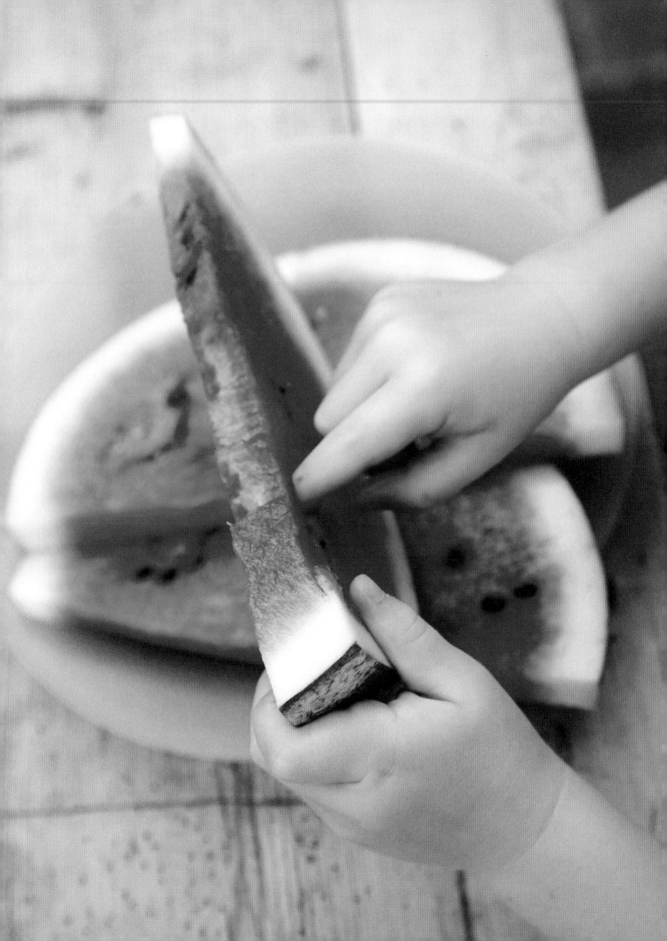

WATERMELON ICE LOLLY

Refreshing, sugar-free ice lollies packed with vitamin A, B, and C are a dream come true especially when they taste this good. Little Allegra is always asking for seconds!

INGREDIENTS

- 2 cups / 300 g watermelon
- 1 heaping cup / 150 g straw-berries
- 1 pear
- 3 tbsp fresh lime juice

PREPARATION

CUT the watermelon into chunks, remove the seeds (or buy seedless watermelon), and put chunks into a large bowl.

RINSE and CUT the leaves off the strawberries and pop into the bowl.

REMOVE the skin off of the pear (make sure you have a very ripe pear) and cut into quarters.

REMOVE its seeds and add to the bowl.

ADD lime juice and mix all ingredients in a blender.

PUT the mixture into ice lolly molds and freeze.

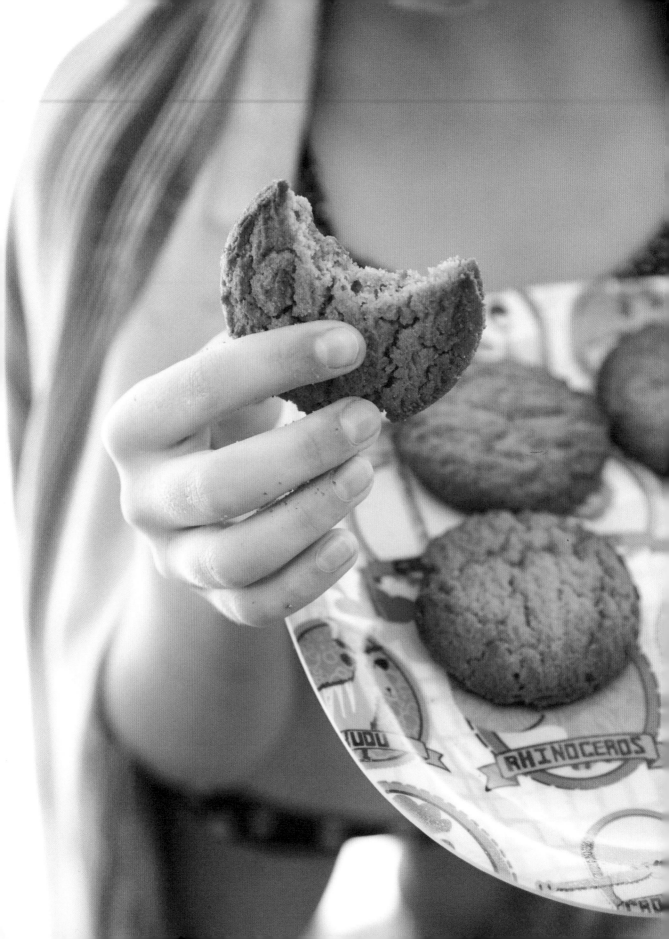

GINGER SNAP COOKIES

A delicious and warming treat, these biscuits satisfy when served on their own or with our Ginger Kiss Tea (see recipe page 26).

INGREDIENTS

- 3 tbsp of grated orange peel
- ¾ tsp fresh grated ginger
- 1 tbsp Manuka honey
- ¼ cup / 55 ml melted coconut oil
- 3 tbsp maple or rice malt syrup
- ¼ cup / 60 g FTF Almond Butter (see recipe page 161)
- ½ cup / 100 g coconut sugar
- ¼ tsp salt
- ½ tsp cinnamon
- ¼ tsp nutmeg (optional)
- 1 ½ cups / 190 g of gluten-free flour
- ½ tsp baking soda
- 1 tbsp white chia seeds

PREPARATION

CARAMELIZE grated orange peel and ginger in a pan over low heat with the honey and 1 teaspoon of water (this should only take a few minutes, and the mixture should not boil).

SET mixture aside and place softened coconut oil, maple or rice malt syrup, almond butter, coconut sugar, salt, and spices in a bowl and beat on a low.

ADD gluten-free flour, baking soda, candied orange peel, and chia seeds, then stir by hand to create a dough. You may need to add up to 1 and ½ cups / 240 to 360 ml of water so that the dough holds its shape and isn't too dry (the chia seeds will expand overnight).

WRAP in cling film and leave the dough to set overnight.

In the morning, PREHEAT oven to 430°F / 220°C.

Carefully ROLL OUT dough, but not too thin as this will cause it to burn. SPRINKLE a little gluten-free flour on the top and cut into shapes.

PLACE on a baking tray lined with baking paper.

BAKE for approximately 10 minutes or until the cookies appear golden brown.

PLACE on a cooling rack before enjoy alone or with complementing ginger tea.

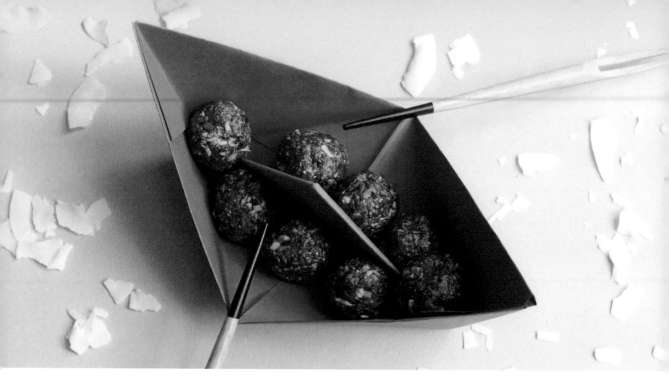

PEANUT BALL BITES

Peanut ball bites contribute to healthy skin and have high vitamin A content, which is an immunity booster. These balls are nutrient-packed, and are also high in antioxidants and protein.

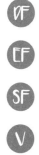

INGREDIENTS

(Makes 12 balls)

- ♣ 2 cups / 180 g oats
- ♣ 1 cup / 250 g FTF Peanut Butter (see recipe page 159)
- ♣ 1 cup / 170 g ground flaxseed
- ♣ 1 cup / 170 g raw chocolate (cut into tiny flakes)
- ♣ 1 cup / 115 g goji berries
- ♣ 1 cup / 130 g pumpkin seeds
- ♣ ⅔ cup / 200 g maple syrup
- ♣ 2 tsp vanilla extract
- ♣ 1 tsp cinnamon

PREPARATION

PUT all the ingredients into a food processor and blend together.

USE your hands to roll mixture into 1 in / 2.5 cm balls.

PUT them into the freezer for 1 hour.

Once they are set, PUT them in the fridge.

WALNUT BALL BITES

High in fiber, walnut ball bites contribute to a healthy digestive system. They are also loaded with minerals such as calcium that help maintain bone health.

INGREDIENTS

(Makes 12 balls)

- ☙ 2 cups / 300 g deseeded Medjool dates
- ☙ 2 tbsp of walnut butter
- ☙ 2 tbsp of ground flaxseed
- ☙ 2 tbsp of orange juice
- ☙ Shredded coconut to coat the ball bites

PREPARATION

PUT all the ingredients but the shredded coconut into a food processor and blend together.

USE your hands to roll mixture into 1 in / 2.5 cm balls.

ROLL balls in shredded coconut.

PUT them into the freezer for 1 hour.

Once they are set, PUT them in the fridge.

CHOCO BALL BITES

High in antioxidants and vitamins such as vitamin A, K, and zinc, these choco balls help promote healthy bones, skin, and a strong heart.

INGREDIENTS

(Makes 12 balls)

- ☙ 1 cup / 150 g deseeded Medjool dates
- ☙ ⅔ cup / 115 g raw dark chocolate
- ☙ ⅔ cup / 110 g chia seeds

PREPARATION

PUT all the ingredients into a food processor and blend together.

USE your hands to roll them into 1 in / 2.5 cm balls.

PUT them into the freezer for 1 hour.

Once they are set, PUT them in the fridge.

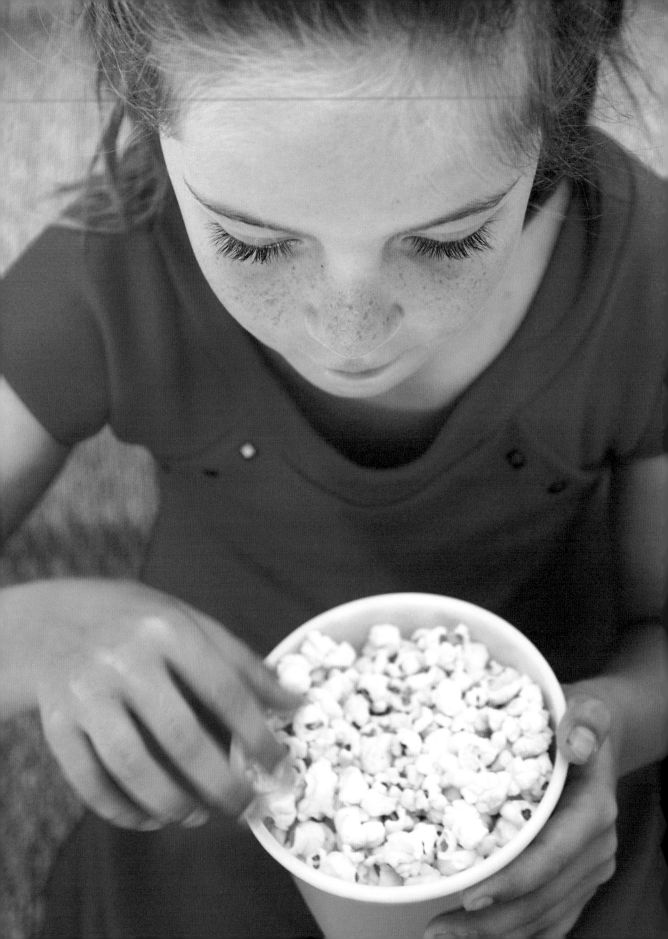

CINNAMON POPCORN

This is Allegra's favorite snack. A scrumptious, light treat perfect for movie nights and parties, this is also an easy snack to pack when on the go! It is filled with fiber and vitamins B and C. Not only will little ones enjoy this yummy treat, but adults will, too!

INGREDIENTS

- 1 cup / 225 g corn kernels
- 1 tsp xylitol
- 1 tsp cinnamon
- 1 tbsp coconut oil
- Extra coconut oil for cooking

PREPARATION

ADD the coconut oil and only a few popcorn kernels to a large pot.

COVER and COOK over medium-high heat until all of the kernels pop, then you will know that the pot is at the correct temperature.

TAKE the popped kernels out of the pot and add the rest of the kernels, arranging them evenly on the pan.

COVER and TAKE the pot off of the heat for 30 seconds. This will heat the kernels, so that they are nearly at popping heat.

PUT the pot back on the heat and the kernels should begin to pop.

SHAKE the pot so that it doesn't burn.

Once the popping slows down, REMOVE the pot and pour the popcorn into a bowl.

In a pan, MELT the coconut oil over low heat and add the cinnamon and xylitol.

ADD the coconut mixture to the popcorn, mixing it thoroughly so that every bite is seasoned.

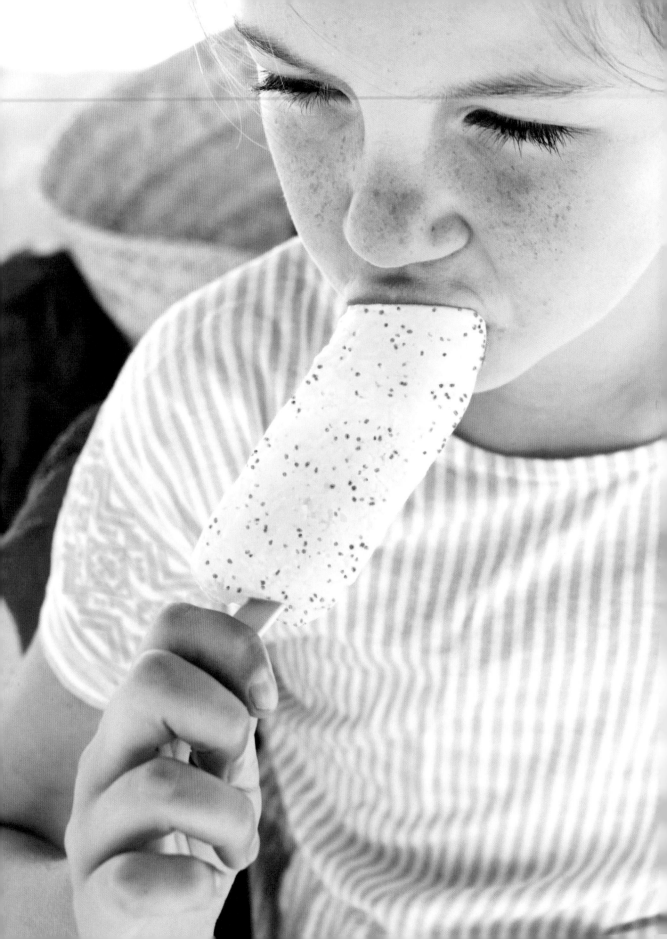

BANANA ORANGE ICE LOLLY

Perfect for a summer afternoon, this hydrating ice lolly will delight while delivering a dose of potassium, omega-3, and vitamin C.

INGREDIENTS

- 1 scant cup / 200 g coconut yogurt
- 2 ripe bananas
- Juice of 2 oranges
- 1 tbsp chia seeds

PREPARATION

ADD the coconut yogurt, banana, and fresh orange juice in a blender and blitz.

MIX in the chia seeds and set aside for a few hours so that they expand.

PLACE the mixture into ice lolly molds and freeze for at least 4 hours.

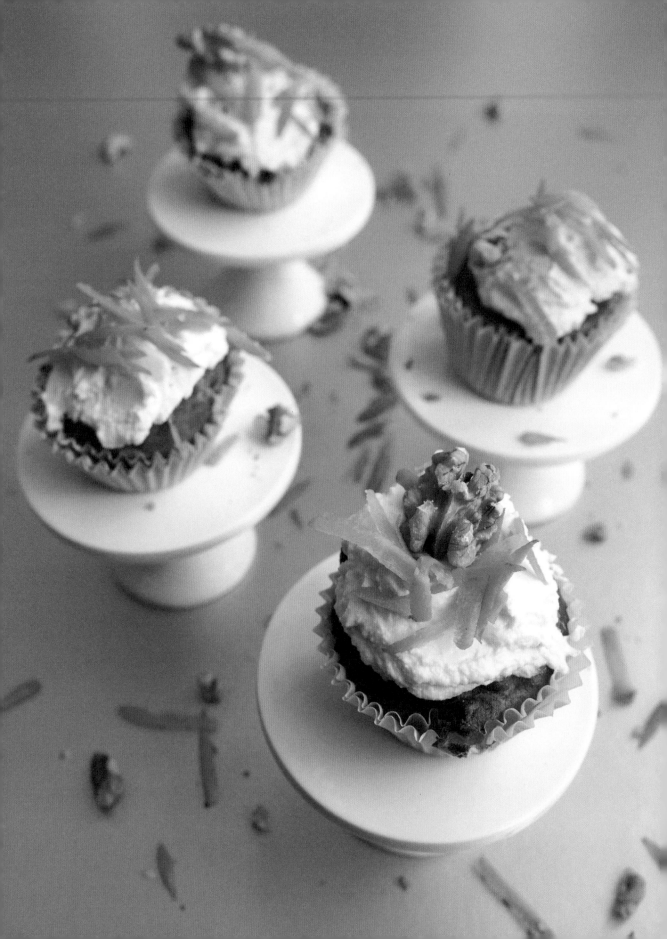

CARROT CUPCAKES

These carrots cupcakes are naturally sweet, we promise your kids will never guess that they're also healthy! This recipe makes for a fun breakfast or dessert.

INGREDIENTS

(Makes 12 cupcakes)

- 1 cup / 120 g of buckwheat flour
- 1 tsp baking soda
- ½ tsp baking powder
- 2 tsp cinnamon
- 1 tsp nutmeg
- 1 pinch sea salt
- 2 eggs
- 1 cup / 240 ml milk of your choice (rice, goat, cow, almond)
- ¼ cup / 100 ml rapeseed oil
- 1 cup / 215 g xylitol
- 2 tsp vanilla extract
- 1 cup / 50 g carrots (grated)
- 1 cup / 90 g desiccated coconut
- 1 cup / 225 g peaches in their natural juice (finely chopped)

Zest of Lemon Frosting:
- 1 ½ cups / 340 g cream cheese
- 3 tbsp agave nectar
- Zest from 1 lemon

PREPARATION

PREHEAT the oven to 350°F / 180°C.

SIFT the flour, baking soda, baking powder, salt, nutmeg, and cinnamon.

In another bowl MIX together the milk, eggs, vanilla extract, oil, and xylitol.

Slowly ADD the dry ingredients and mix well.

COMBINE the carrots, coconut, some lemon zest, and peaches in another bowl, then slowly add to the mixture.

POUR the mixture into cupcake cases and bake for 10 to 15 minutes or until golden brown.

Once the cupcakes are in the oven, start MAKING the frosting.

COMBINE the cream cheese, lemon zest, and agave nectar, then mix well.

Once the cupcakes are out of the oven and have cooled, gently SPREAD the frosting on top and serve.

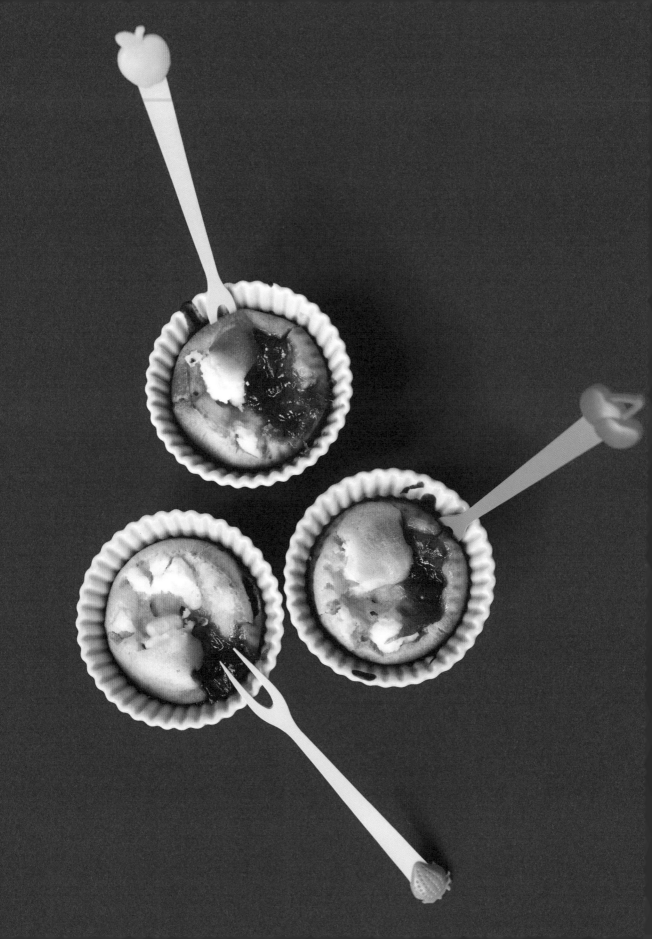

BERRY CHEESECAKE MUFFINS

The muffins are filled with protein and make a wholesome snack.

INGREDIENTS

(Makes 6 muffins)

- 1 ¾ cups / 220 g coconut flour
- 2 eggs (lightly beaten)
- 3 tbsp coconut oil
- ½ cup / 170 g coconut suger
- 2 tbsp of FTF Raw Berry Jam (see recipe page 160)
- ¼ cup / 60 g coconut yogurt
- ⅓ cup / 110 ml maple syrup
- ¼ cup / 60 g ricotta

PREPARATION

PREHEAT the oven to 350°F / 180°C.

Lightly GREASE six muffin holders with coconut oil.

PLACE the oil, coconut sugar, yogurt, maple syrup, and eggs into a bowl and combine.

ADD the flour and mix the batter until combined.

SPOON mixture into the muffin holders, only filling ¾ of the tin.

ADD a scoop of ricotta and jam to each muffin, then cover with a small amount of batter.

BAKE for 30 minutes or until lightly golden.

ALLOW to cool before enjoying.

GF

PF

SF

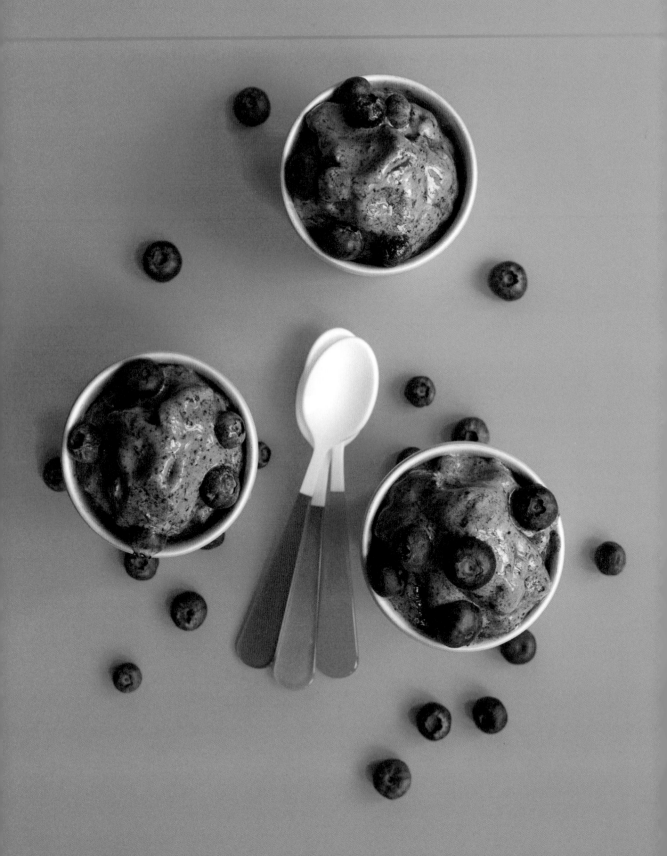

BABA'S FROYO

Froyo is definitely an old favorite, not to mention one of the healthiest and most simple desserts. It is easy to make and a tasty treat. We hope you enjoy it as much as we do!

INGREDIENTS

- 1 ½ cup / 200 g frozen blueberries
- 1 scant cup / 225 g Greek or coconut yogurt
- 1 tsp xylitol

PREPARATION

Sometimes keeping it simple makes the best recipes. This is the easiest recipe in the world. All you need to do is MIX all these ingredients into a blender and serve it up!

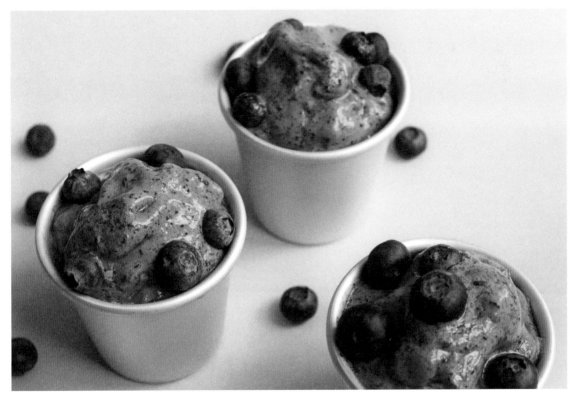

SAVORY SNACKS

Kids love snacks and we consider them a great way
to give children nutritious goodness between meals
so their energy levels don't drop. Eating is also great
for their sensory skills and picking at food makes eating
fun for them. Here are some delicious snacks we have
come up with for the little ones (and everyone else) to enjoy.

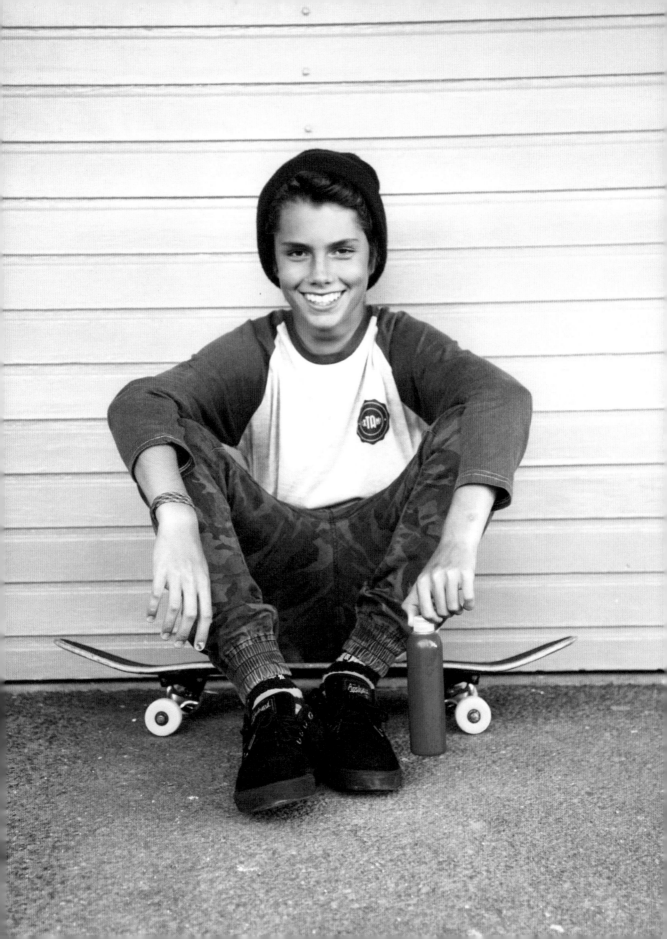

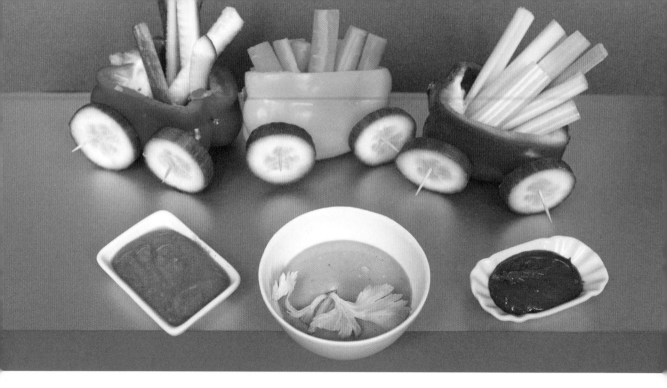

DIP TRAIN

The Dip Train is an edible centerpiece for parties and a fun way to sneak plenty of vegetables and protein into your kid's diets. There are so many healthy hidden ingredients in these dips. Choose as many as you like to make it a large or small train.

GREEN PEA DIP

This dip is a perfect way to get in some rich phyto-nutrients, minerals, and antioxidants into your little ones.

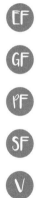

INGREDIENTS

* 1 cup / 170 g peas
* 1 tbsp cilantro (chopped)
* 2 tbsp tahini
* 1 tbsp water
* 1 tbsp lemon juice
* Salt and pepper to taste

PREPARATION

SET aside a small amount of the peas.

PLACE the rest of the ingredients in a blender and pulse until mixture relatively is smooth.

ADD remaining peas and blend slightly for a chunkier consistency.

BEET HUMMUS DIP

This delicious dip is immune system boosting, memory improving, and antioxidant rich. The whole family is dipping for more goodness.

INGREDIENTS

* 2 medium sized beets (skin on)
* 1 can chickpeas
* 2 cloves garlic
* 3 tbsp tahini
* 1 tbsp lemon juice
* Salt to taste
* Filtered water to thin

PREPARATION

PREHEAT oven to 340°F / 170°C.

WRAP each beet individually in foil and roast in the oven for about 2 hours, or until soft and tender.

Once beets are roasted, REMOVE them from the oven and let cool.

PEEL skin and chop into chunks.

DRAIN, RINSE, and SKIN the chickpeas.

MIX beets, chickpeas, and garlic in a food processor for 1 minute.

ADD lemon juice, tahini, and salt and continue mixing.

Slowly ADD water to the blending mixture until hummus becomes creamy and smooth.

REFRIGERATE or serve immediately.

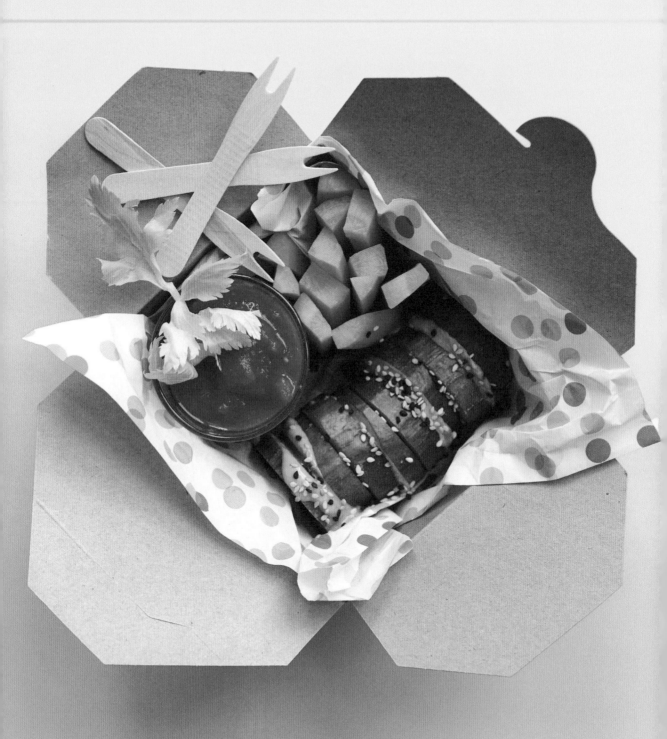

BEAN DIP

This dip is great with oat crackers, veggies, crostini, or tortilla chips. Beans are very filling and kidney beans in particular are high in fiber. That fiber helps prevent insulin levels from rising too quickly making this a great snack for diabetic kids. This snack is also high in protein, vitamin B1, manganese, iron, potassium, and magnesium.

INGREDIENTS

* 1 ¼ cup / 400 g canned kidney beans (drained and rinsed)
* 2 tbsp capers
* 2 tbsp olive oil
* 2 tbsp lemon juice
* 1 tsp lime juice
* 2 tsp Dijon mustard
* 1 garlic clove
* Paprika and olive oil for garnish

PREPARATION

RINSE and DRAIN the beans in a sieve and put into a food processor.

ADD capers, lemon and lime juice, garlic, and mustard to the food processor and blend together.

GARNISH with olive oil and paprika for a bit of color.

ARTICHOKE DIP

On the dip train, we have also included this super dip that is high in fiber, antioxidants, and supplies your body with digestive support as well as a brain boost! We should actually call this the Superhero Dip.

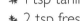

INGREDIENTS

* 1 ¼ cup / 400 g canned cannellini beans (drained and rinsed)
* 1 ¾ cup / 400 g canned artichoke hearts (drained)
* 1 tsp tahini
* 2 tsp fresh lemon juice
* 1 tsp fresh lime juice
* 1 garlic clove (crushed)
* 1 pinch red pepper flakes
* ¼ cup / 50 ml extra virgin olive oil
* Salt and pepper to taste
* Parsley (minced) for garnish

PREPARATION

PLACE the cannellini beans, artichoke hearts, tahini, lemon juice, lime juice, garlic, and red pepper flakes in a food processor and blend until fairly smooth.

With the motor still running, slowly DRIZZLE in the olive oil.

SEASON to taste with salt and pepper.

SERVE at room temperature or chilled with some minced parsley for garnish.

GUACAMOLE DIP

This all-time favorite is a creamy dip the kids will be fighting over. It is packed full of goodness like vitamins K, E, and C. It works well as a veggie dip, on Super Seed Crackers (see recipe page 76), or even with a chicken or salmon dish.

INGREDIENTS

* 3 ripe avocados
* ½ lemon
* ¼ red onion (chopped)
* 1 bunch fresh cilantro
* 1 ripe tomato (deseeded and finely sliced)

PREPARATION

PEEL and PIT avocados, then place in a bowl and mash with a fork.

SQUEEZE some lemon on the avocado and place to the side.

GUACAMOLE DIP

- ❋ 2 limes freshly juiced
- ❋ Extra virgin olive oil
- ❋ Sea salt

PLACE onion, cilantro, lime juice, olive oil, and tomato slices into a blender and pulse.

COMBINE onion mixture into the avocado mash and add sea salt to taste.

VEGAN CREPES

These multi-purpose crepes are great, especially when you're on the go. You can use them to make a sweet snack by adding "Un-Nutella" (see recipe page 36) or you can use them to make a savory wrap. We often put chicken, mashed avocado, cucumber, and tomatoes inside.

INGREDIENTS

- ❋ 1 cup / 240 ml Oat Milk (see recipe page 21)
- ❋ 1 tbsp fresh lemon juice
- ❋ 1 cup gluten-free all-purpose flour
- ❋ ¼ tsp salt

PREPARATION

SIFT the flour and salt into a large bowl.

WHISK the oat milk in a small bowl.

MAKE a hole in the center of the dry ingredients and pour in oat milk and lemon juice.

BLEND the mixture together (it will be lumpy).

HEAT a lightly oiled pan over medium-high heat.

DROP the batter into the pan with a large spoon.

COOK until bubbles form and the edges are dry.

FLIP and COOK until browned on the other side.

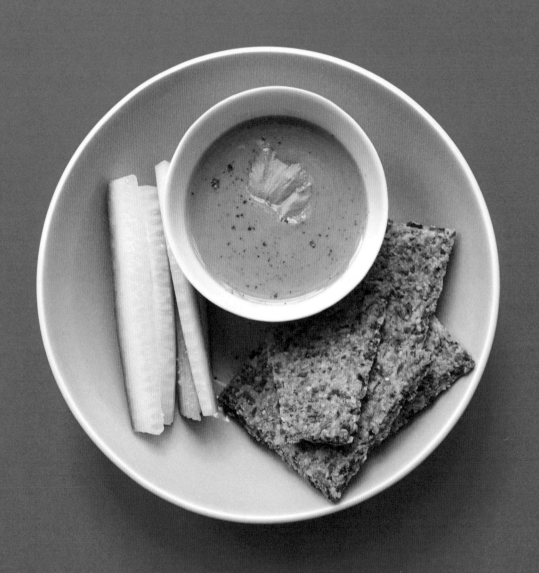

SUPER SEED CRACKERS

These crackers are filled with omegas! Enjoy them alone or with your choice of dips (see recipes pages 70 to 74).

INGREDIENTS

* ½ cup / 70 g pumpkin seeds
* ½ cup / 90 g flaxseeds
* ½ cup / 80 g sesame seeds
* ½ cup / 80 g chia seeds
* ½ cup / 70 g almond meal (or blended almonds)
* 1 cup / 240 ml filtered water
* Salt (or cinnamon for sweet crackers)

PREPARATION

PREHEAT oven to 325°F / 160°C.

LINE a baking tray with nonstick paper.

PLACE all ingredients into a blender and combine.

SPREAD the mixture thinly on the baking trays and place in oven.

BAKE for 40 minutes, or until crisp.

TAKE the crackers out of the oven and break up.

SPRINKLE with either salt or cinnamon, then cook the other side for an additional 15 minutes.

REMOVE from oven and allow to cool.

SERVE or STORE in an airtight container.

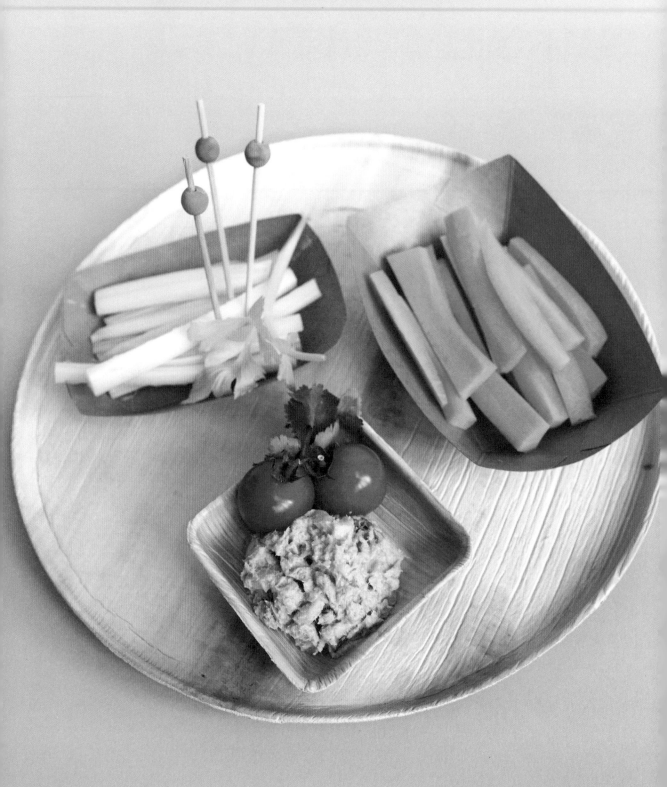

MACKEREL & SARDINE PATE

This dish is an omega-3 heaven. Sardines and mackerel are high in the good fats that are great for healthy-looking skin, helping to control blood sugar levels, and lowering bad cholesterol. This pate works great on rye bread or store-bought gluten-free crackers.

INGREDIENTS

* 12 oz / 350 g mackerel (fresh or canned in water)
* 1.7 oz / 50 g sardines (canned)
* ⅓ cup / 70 ml extra virgin olive oil
* Juice of 3 lemons
* ½ cucumber (finely sliced)
* 1 tbsp Dijon mustard
* 1 pinch smoked paprika

PREPARATION

If you are using fresh mackerel, POACH the mackerel. PLACE the fillets into a wide pan with ½ cup / 100 ml of water. BRING water up to a simmer and cook for 3 to 5 minutes. REMOVE mackerel from the pan and let it cool on a plate.

REMOVE the mackerel skin and add both fish to the blender.

ADD Dijon mustard, smoked paprika, extra virgin olive oil, and lemon juice, then blend until smooth.

ADD the finely sliced cucumber into the mixture.

We don't normally add salt as the lemons and sardines give this dish a salty taste, but if you want to add some sea salt, please do!

LUNCH

Lunchtime can be a slippery slope as kids have a lot of control over what they eat. When they are at school, and unsupervised, they can choose to eat the healthy items that their parents pack, or discard them. This makes teaching kids about the importance of eating a healthy lunch even more important.

Breakfast is the fuel that gets kids' engines running, and lunch is their top-up fuel. Children who put the wrong type of fuel into their tanks can run out of energy before the day is over, whereas who children fuel up right will continue to cruise all afternoon.

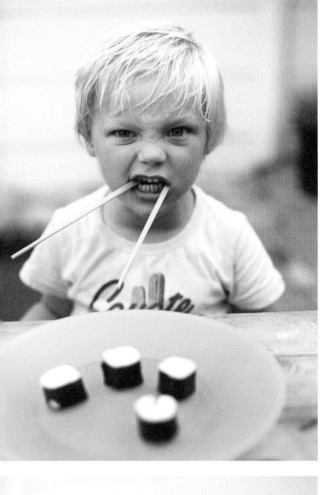
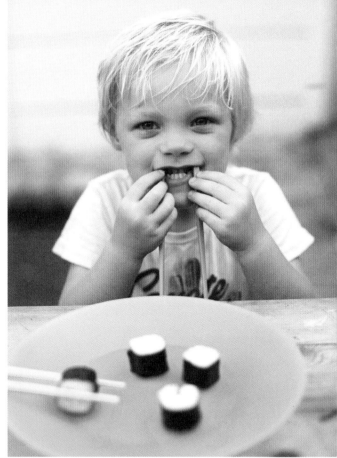
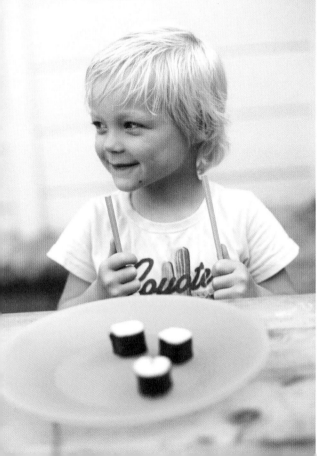
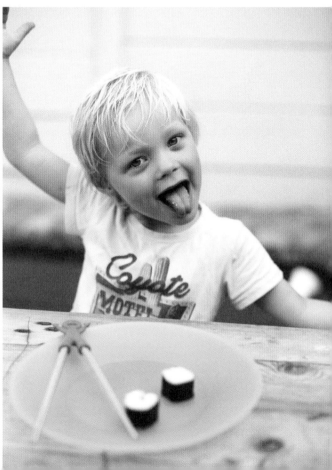

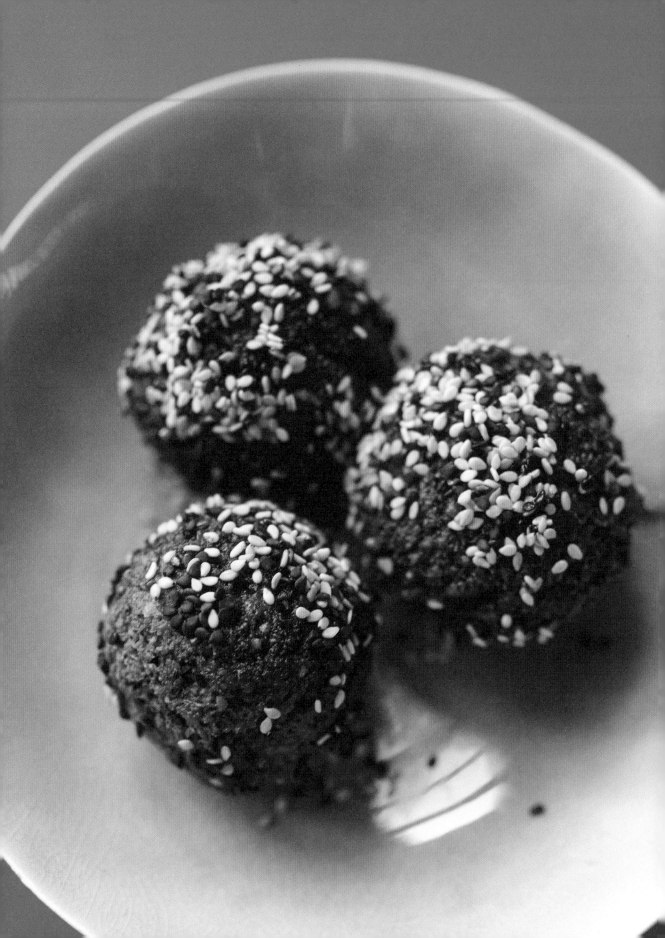

KIMIA'S FALAFELS

Filled with iron and protein, these falafels make for a fantastic vegetarian lunch option.

INGREDIENTS

- 2 ¼ cups / 400 g brown lentils (drained and rinsed if canned)
- ⅔ cup / 70 g gluten-free breadcrumbs (we like using rice or almond, or try making your own by roughly blending gluten-free bread)
- 1 tsp cumin
- ⅜ cup / 100 g coconut yogurt or ricotta
- ⅓ cup / 5 g cilantro leaves
- 1 tsp lemon rind
- 1 egg
- Coconut oil
- White and black sesame seeds
- Salt and pepper to taste

PREPARATION

PREHEAT oven to 425°F / 220°C.

PLACE the lentils, gluten-free breadcrumbs, ricotta or coconut yogurt, egg, cumin, cilantro, lemon rind, and salt in a food processor and pulse until everything is combined.

SHAPE into small balls and brush with coconut oil.

ROLL the balls in the black and white sesame seeds.

PLACE on a baking tray lined with nonstick paper.

BAKE for 10 minutes, or until crisp.

SERVE with Beet Hummus Dip (see recipe page 71) and quinoa or salad.

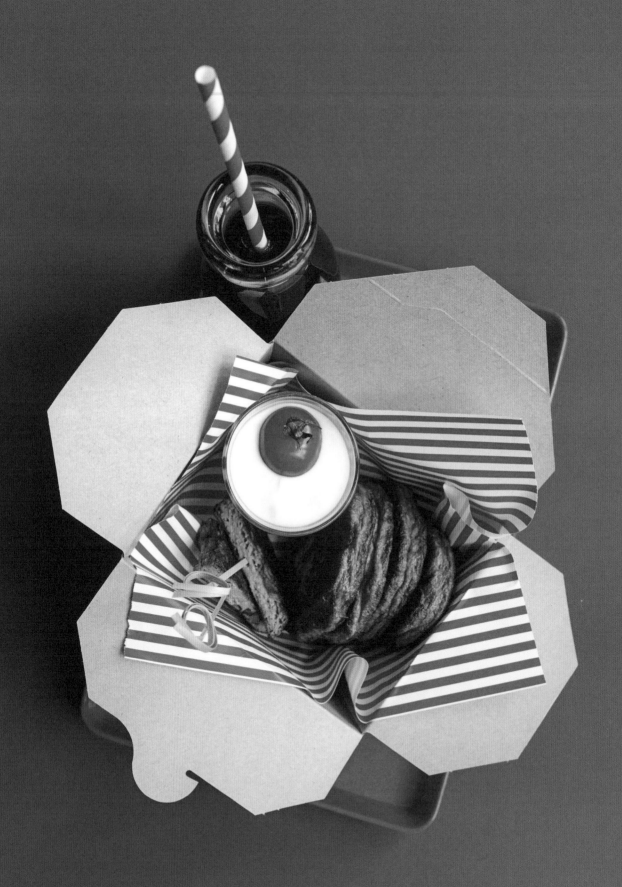

GREEN FRITTERS

Who knew fritters could be so good? The future grand-prix champion Rex loves this yummy green dish. It is a great way to pack in protein and all those leafy greens. Here we have iron, phosphorus, and zinc giving kids the fuel they need to concentrate and learn, as well as increasing their stamina to play. This is also an easy dish to bring with you when you are on the move.

INGREDIENTS

- 3 cups / 500 g green peas
- 1 small bunch baby spinach
- ¼ ripe avocado
- 1 cup / 140 g gluten-free corn flour
- 2 eggs
- Coconut oil

PREPARATION

BLANCH peas and baby spinach for 10 seconds in boiling water, strain and cool.

ADD the peas, baby spinach, avocado, corn flour, and eggs in a food processor.

In a hot nonstick pan, ADD coconut oil and fry about ½ cup / 110 g of pea mix until golden brown.

If you have a star-shaped cookie cutter, PLACE this on the fry pan and pour in mixture to create a fun-shaped fritter.

FLIP over and repeat on the other side.

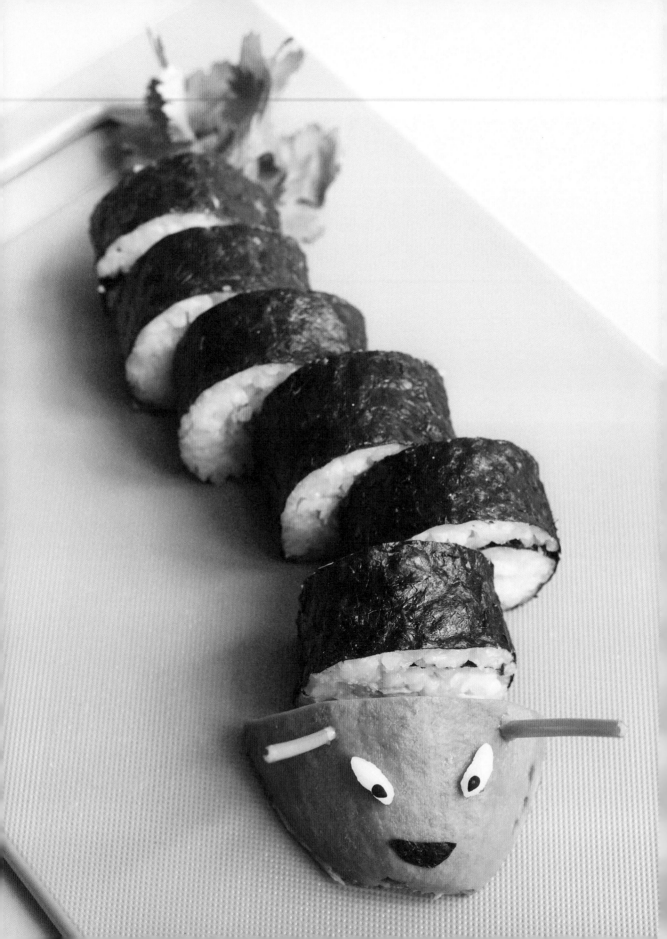

AVOCADO TUNA ROLL

Kids love sushi rolls! They are a fun meal or snack. Choose from our different fillings and rice options.

INGREDIENTS

- 1.5 oz / 40 g glass jar of tuna in olive oil
- ¼ ripe avocado
- Lemon wedge
- 1 nori sheet
- ⅓ cup / 80 g sushi rice (cooked)

PREPARATION

MASH up the tuna and mix in the avocado.

SEASON with a small amount of salt and a squeeze of lemon.

CUT the nori paper into ⅔ of a piece.

PLACE the nori paper on a sushi mat.

PUT a thin layer of cooked rice on the nori paper, leaving space at the end of the paper.

PRESS the rice firmly into the nori paper.

ADD the avocado and tuna mixture in a line down the center.

LIFT the side of the mat and roll to seal the edges.

USE your hands to roll the shape and properly seal the cylinder shape of the sushi roll.

With a sharp knife, CUT the roll into 0.5 in / 2 cm slices.

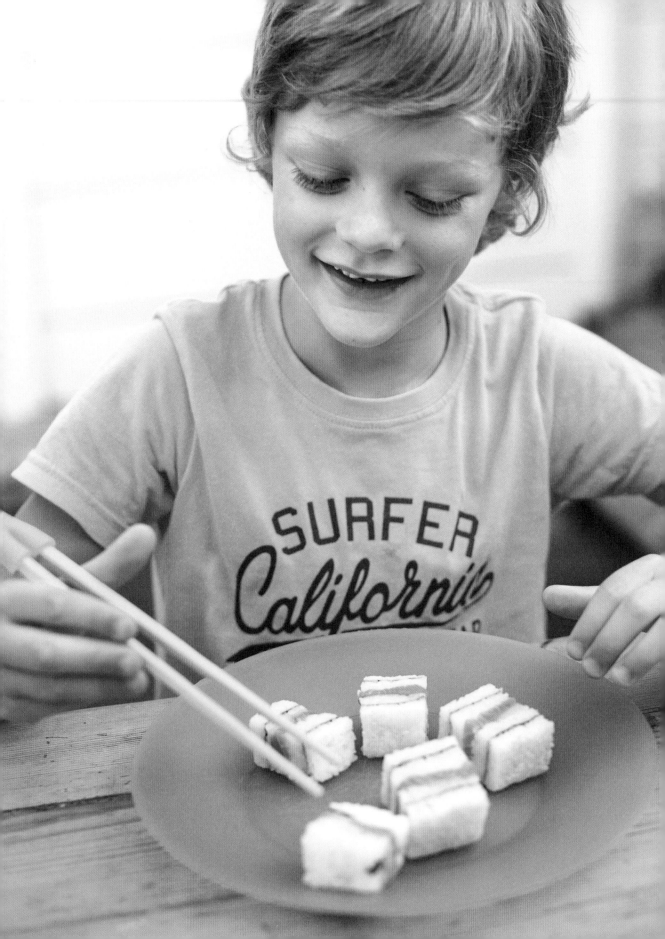

AVOCADO SALMON ROLL

This is brain food wrapped in antioxidant heaven. Goodness has never looked so cool!
This is Waldorf's favorite dish, he calls them his "ninja rolls."

INGREDIENTS

- 1 fillet of salmon
- Small amount of honey
- ¼ ripe avocado
- Lemon wedge
- 1 nori sheet
- ⅓ cup / 80 g sushi rice (cooked)

PREPARATION

TURN the oven onto grill at high.

Lightly GLAZE the salmon with a small amount of honey (optional).

COOK salmon in the oven for 7 minutes until the fish is lightly cooked.

SET aside to cool.

CUT the nori paper into ⅔ of a piece.

PLACE the nori paper on a sushi mat.

PUT a thin layer of rice on the nori paper, leaving space at the end of the paper.

PRESS the rice firmly into the nori paper.

ADD pieces of flaked salmon and pieces of avocado in a line down the center.

LIFT the side of the mat and roll to seal the edges.

USE your hands to roll the shape and properly seal the cylinder shape of the sushi roll.

With a sharp knife, CUT the roll into 0.5 in / 2 cm slices.

AVOCADO CUCUMBER ROLL

This light cucumber roll is vegan and one of Tali's favorites. Not only delicious, it fills the body with vitamins and minerals.

INGREDIENTS

- 1 nori sheet
- ⅓ cup / 80 g sushi rice (cooked)
- ¼ ripe avocado
- Lemon wedge
- 2 small carrots (peeled and sliced into long, very thin pieces)
- 1 cucumber (peeled and sliced into very long pieces)
- FTF Mayonnaise (optional) (see recipe page 161)

PREPARATION

CUT the nori paper into ⅔ of a piece. Place the nori paper on a sushi mat.

PUT a thin layer of cooked rice on the nori paper, leaving space at the end of the paper.

PRESS the rice firmly into the nori paper.

ADD slices of avocado (squeezing lemon on the avocado), cucumber, and carrots in a line down the center of the roll.

DRIZZLE mayonnaise onto the vegetables (optional).

LIFT the side of the mat and roll to seal the edges.

USE your hands to roll the shape and properly seal the cylinder shape of the sushi roll.

With a sharp knife, CUT the roll into 0.5 in / 2 cm slices.

COD FISH FINGERS WITH COCONUT

All kids love fish fingers, they are easy to make and easy to eat and packed with Omega 3, protein, and energy.

INGREDIENTS

- 1 tbsp desiccated coconut
- 1 tbsp rice flour
- 1 tbsp gluten-free bread-crumbs
- 1 tbsp flaxseeds (ground)
- ½ tsp salt
- 1 ½ cup / ⅛ pint Oat Milk (see recipe page 21)
- 1 tbsp maple syrup
- 21 oz / 600 g skinless, boneless cod
- Rapeseed oil for cooking
- Rock salt for seasoning

PREPARATION

MIX together the desiccated coconut, rice flour, breadcrumbs, flaxseeds, and salt in a medium-large sized bowl.

MIX together the oat milk and maple syrup in a separate medium-large sized bowl.

CUT cod into small strips (approximately the width of two fingers and the length of your index finger). Make sure there are no bones.

PUT wax paper on a baking tray and turn the oven on grill to high.

TAKE the pieces of fish and dip them into the wet mixture.

Once the fish is coated, ROLL it into the dry mixture, making sure that every side is covered.

PLACE fish fingers on the baking tray and drizzle them with a small amount of rapeseed oil.

GRILL for 5 to 7 minutes until lightly golden and fish is tender.

SEASON with rock salt.

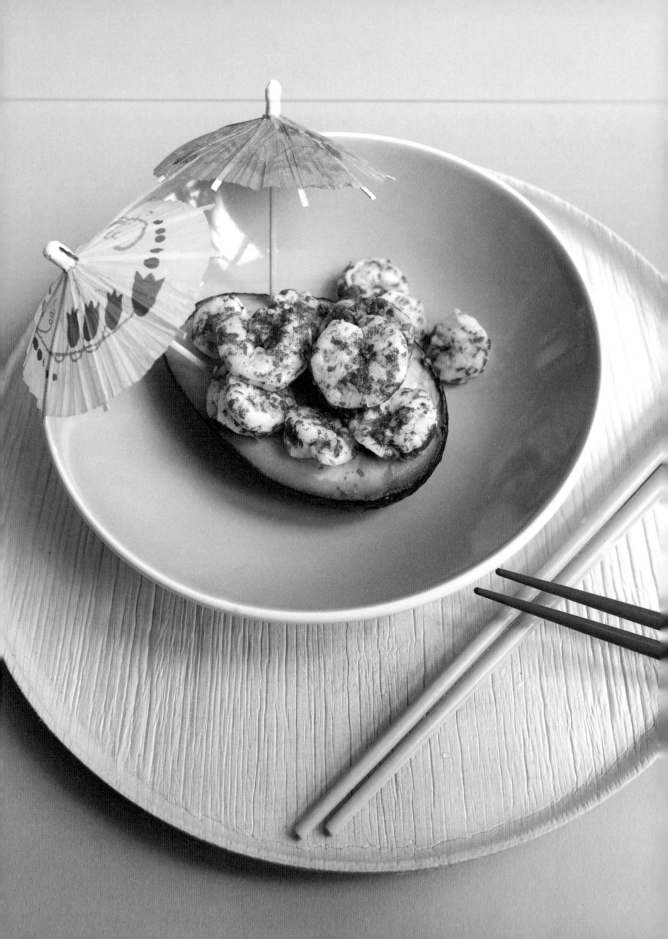

AVOCADO & SHRIMP

This was Lohralee's favorite dish when she was a little girl. Her dad used to make it for her and now she makes it for her children. This snack is high in anti-inflammatory and antioxidant properties such as vitamin E, selenium, and copper. The vitamin B12 in this dish also helps with brain function so your kids will be as clever as can be!

INGREDIENTS

- 1 handful of cilantro
- Juice of 2 limes
- 5.3 oz / 150 g baby shrimp (cooked)
- 1 tbsp extra virgin olive oil
- 1 ripe avocado

PREPARATION

ADD the lime juice and cilantro into a food processor and blend together until they become a paste.

PUT the paste into a bowl and mix in the extra virgin olive oil, then the baby shrimp.

CUT avocado in half.

PLACE mixture on top of each avocado half and voilà, you are all set to go!

SOUPS & STEWS

*Soups and stews are warming and nourishing.
They can retain more nutrients than conventional cooking
and are great on their own or as a starter for a hearty meal.
We particularly love feeding soups and stews to children
as they are easy to digest for little bodies.*

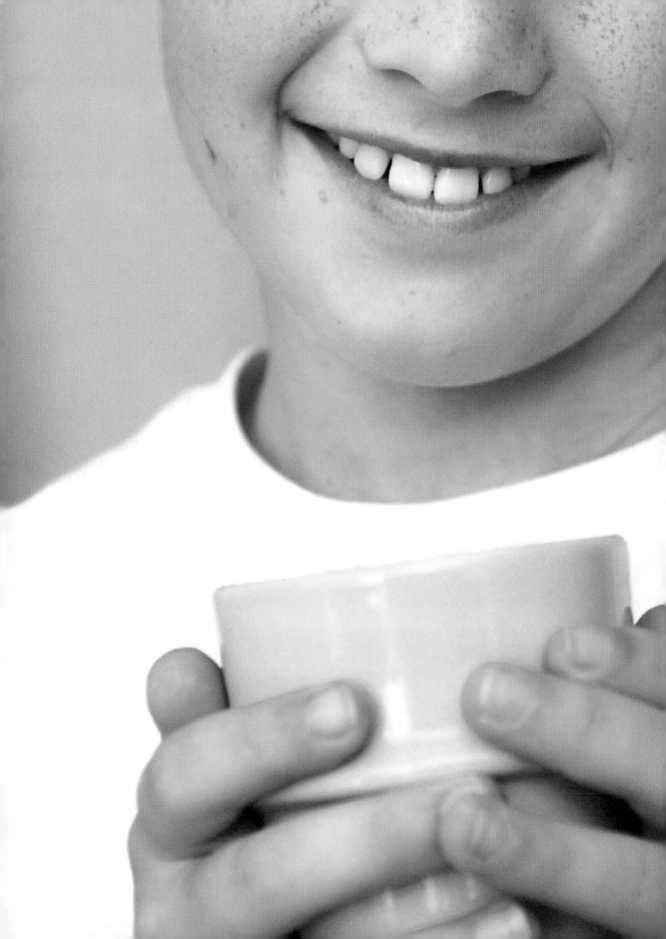

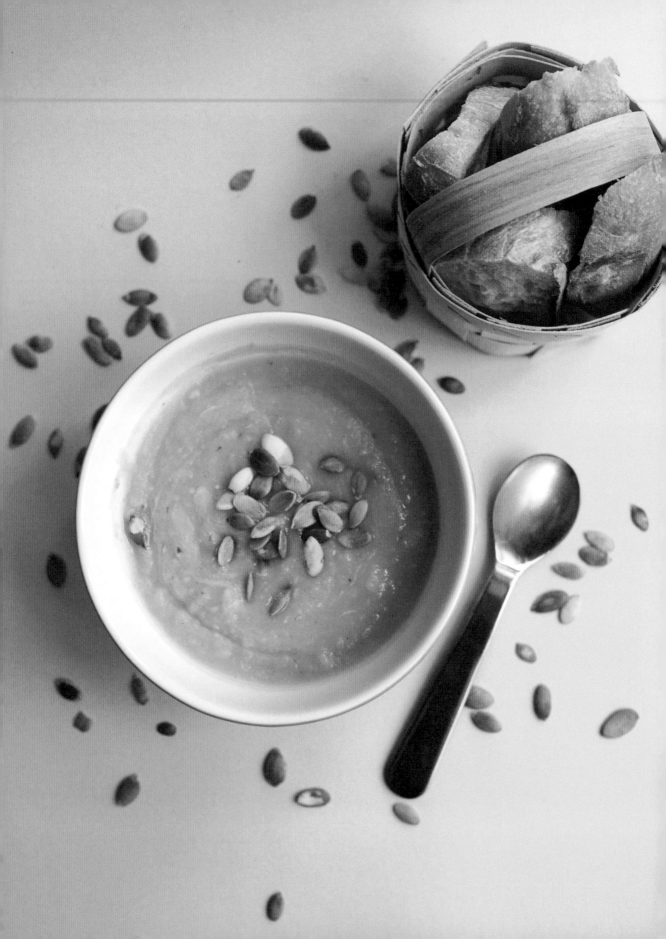

ESTI & GEKKO'S PUMPKIN SOUP

This recipe is a favorite of our little friends Estelle (7) and Gekko (5). They love it on chilly days after school, as well as for dinner. Their mummy Julia makes it for them regularly.

INGREDIENTS

- 1 Hokkaido pumpkin
- 1 medium onion
  (cut into small cubes)
- 1 cup / 250 ml filtered
  water
- 1.5–2 oz / 50–70 g ginger
  (grated)
- 1 tsp curry powder
- 1 tsp cumin
- 1 tsp coconut sugar
- Himalayan pink rock salt
  and pepper to taste
- 1 handful pumpkin seeds
  (optional)

PREPARATION

CUT the pumpkin into 0.5 in / 1.5 cm to 2 cm chunks, keeping the peel on, but removing the seeds.

Lightly FRY the onion cubes in olive oil, then put to the side.

BRING filtered water to a boil.

ADD in the onion, pumpkin, grated ginger, curry powder, cumin, and coconut sugar.

COOK for 20 minutes on medium heat, then puree the mixture.

SEASON with salt and pepper to taste.

If you would like a creamier texture, ADD some oat cream.

GARNISH with some pumpkin seeds (optional).

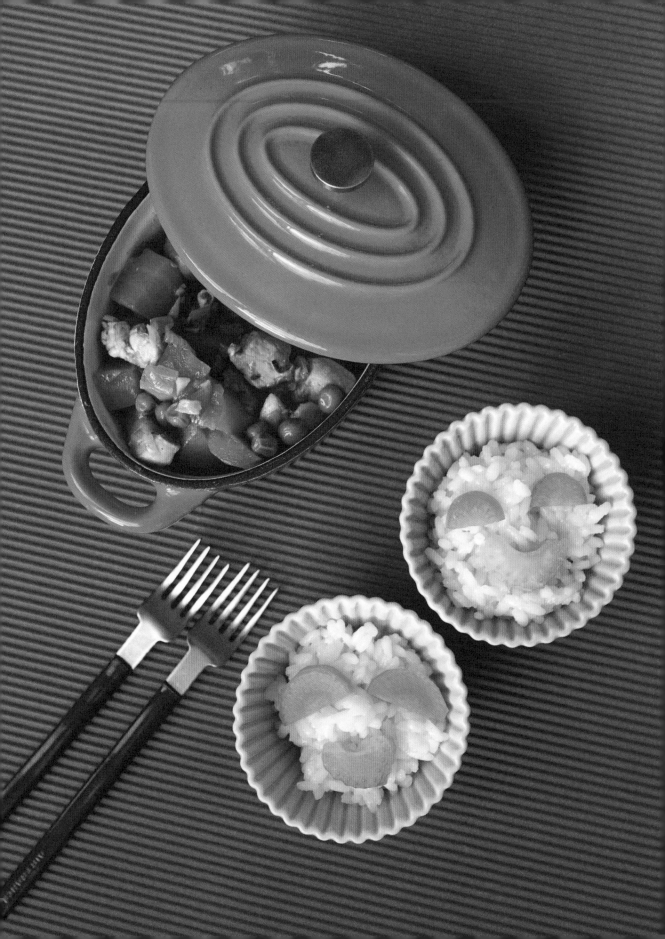

CHICKEN STEW

This is one of Waldorf's favorites as he loves chicken. It's a slow cook meal, so you can just pop all the ingredients into a pot, leave it for 45 minutes, and voilà! You have a yummy scrummy dish.

INGREDIENTS

- 14 oz / 400 g chicken thighs or breast
- 2 wheat-free sausages
- 1 ½ onion (finely chopped)
- 1 garlic (finely chopped)
- 2 carrots (cut into bite-sized pieces)
- 1 ½ cup / 250 g peas
- 2 heaping cups / 500 ml chicken stock
- 6 new baby potatoes

PREPARATION

EMPTY the sausages out of their cases into a large pot.

COOK the sausages for 2 to 3 minutes at medium heat until some of the juicy fat comes out of the sausage.

ADD the chopped garlic and onions and cook for another 2 to 3 minutes, or until they have softened.

ADD the chicken thighs and cook until the chicken is no longer pink.

Once the chicken is lightly cooked on both sides, ADD the chicken stock, peas, carrots, and potatoes.

SET the stovetop temperature to the lowest possible setting, put the pot lid on, and cook for 30 to 45 minutes.

When the chicken stew is ready to serve, CUT the new baby potatoes in half, add a little butter or olive oil, and enjoy!

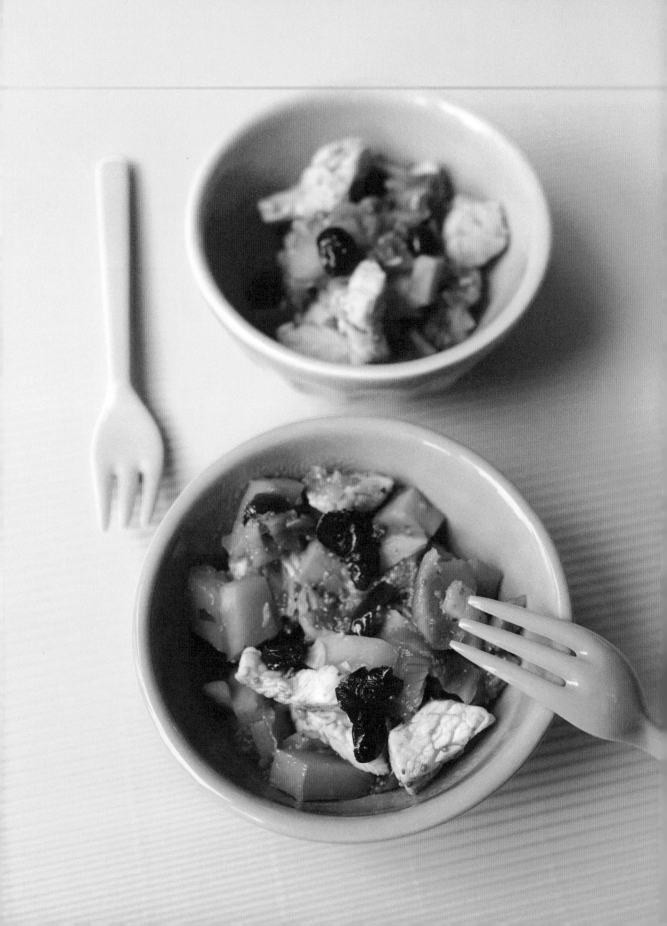

TURKEY STEW

*The combination of turkey with cranberries and figs gives this tasty stew a sweet holiday feel.
Turkey is easily digested, low in fat, and high in protein which is very important for children's growth.
Cranberries, sweet potatoes, and butternut squash are filled with antioxidants and have
anti-inflammatory properties.*

INGREDIENTS

- 1 onion (finely chopped)
- 2 cloves of garlic
  (finely chopped)
- 7 oz / 500 g turkey
  (cut into chunks)
- 1 cup / 240 ml turkey stock
- 6 dried figs
  (finely chopped)
- 1 handful of frozen cranberries (finely chopped)
- ½ cup / 75 g butternut
  squash or pumpkin
  (chopped)
- ½ cup / 75 g sweet potato
  (chopped)
- Coconut oil

PREPARATION

GREASE the bottom of a medium sized pot
with coconut oil.

Once the coconut oil has melted, ADD the finely chopped
garlic cloves and onion and cook for 2 minutes.

Once the color of the onions becomes translucent,
ADD the turkey chunks and cook until
they become white.

ADD the turkey stock, figs, and cranberries
with the butternut squash and sweet potato.

This dish should be cooked on low/simmer
for 30 to 45 minutes.

BEEF STEW

Nothing beats comfort food, especially when it is packed with goodness. Stews are a great way to get all the nutrients you need without losing any nutritional value. You'll also notice the kids coming back for seconds…

INGREDIENTS

- 2 lbs / 900 g beef chuck roast (cut into ½ in / 1 cm cubes)
- 3 tbsp olive oil
- 2 cups / 300 g carrots (sliced)
- 2 celery stalks (sliced)
- 2 cups potatoes
- 1 large onion
- 4 garlic cloves (minced)
- 27 oz / 800 g canned diced tomatoes
- 4 cups / 1 l water
- 1 tbsp cider vinegar
- 1 tsp Italian seasoning
- 2 tbsp parsley (minced)
- Salt and pepper to taste

PREPARATION

COMBINE (stew or shin) beef cubes in a large bowl.

In a medium saucepan over medium-high heat, SAUTÉ beef in oil stirring occasionally until beef is slightly browned, 5 to 10 minutes. (Beef will not cook entirely.)

PLACE beef in a 3 qt / 2.8 l slow cooker.

ADD carrots, celery, potatoes, onion, garlic, tomatoes, water, vinegar, and seasonings.

STIR to combine and cook beef stew on low heat for 5 to 6 hours.

SEASON with salt, pepper, and parsley before serving.

CARROT SOUP

Filled with vitamin C and beta carotene, this soup may just help you see better at night as the old wives' tale goes!

INGREDIENTS

- 1 lb / 450 g carrots (peeled and sliced)
- 1 onion (chopped)
- 1 garlic clove (crushed)
- 1 tsp ground cilantro
- 1 lemon (juiced)
- 1 lime (juiced)
- 1 tsp nutmeg
- 8.5 oz / 250 ml oat cream
- 1 tbsp vegetable oil
- 1.5 qt / 1.5 l vegetable stock
- 1 handful fresh cilantro (chopped)
- Coconut oil

PREPARATION

HEAT the coconut oil in a large pan.

ADD vegetables and sauté for 3 to 5 minutes, or until they are beginning to soften.

STIR in the seasoning and cook for a couple of minutes.

ADD the vegetable stock and bring to a boil, cover and simmer for about 35 minutes, or until the carrots are tender.

LET the soup cool down then blend, adding the oat cream.

GARNISH with fresh cilantro.

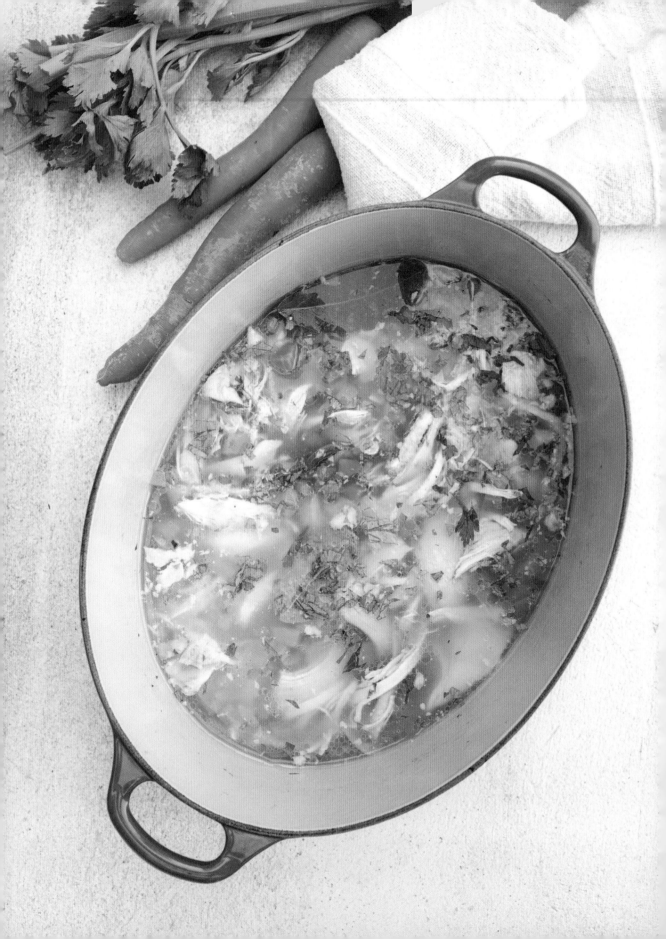

NANA'S CHICKEN SOUP

Perfect when your kids are feeling under the weather, chicken soup is a traditional cure for an array of ailments. Filled with protein, vitamins, and nutrients, this soup proves Nana knew best!

INGREDIENTS

- 1 whole chicken
- 1 medium yellow onion (chopped)
- 4 carrots (chopped)
- 1 parsnip (chopped)
- 2 potatoes
- 3 cloves garlic (crushed)
- 2 stalks celery (chopped)
- 2 tsp sea salt
- 1 tsp whole peppercorns
- 1 bay leaf
- 1 handful parsley (finely chopped)
- 1 handful thyme (finely chopped)

"Veggies for Later":
- 4 carrots (finely chopped)
- 1 cup / 170 g peas
- 1 potato (finely chopped)

PREPARATION

PUT all of the ingredients into the biggest pot you have.

FILL pot to the top with filtered water until all ingredients are covered with 1 in / 2.5 cm of liquid.

PUT on the lid and COOK on low until the water begins to boil. This should take about 30 to 45 minutes.

OPEN the lid a bit so the steam can escape from the pot (we put a wooden spoon between the pot and the lid to prop it open).

COOK for another 30 minutes.

REMOVE the soup from the heat and take the chicken out of the pot. PUT it on a large plate and let it cool.

STRAIN and keep the broth, setting aside the cooked vegetables.

PUT the broth back into the pot, ADD the "Veggies for Later," and cook for 15 minutes.

Once the chicken has cooled down, PICK all the meat off of the bones and add it to the soup.

With the left over cooked vegetables, you can create a veggie mash side dish for the kids.

DINNER

Dinner is a wonderful opportunity for parents to sit down with their children and enjoy quality family time. Not only is a healthy, nutrient-rich dinner literally brain food, the conversation that adults have with children in a relaxed environment at the table will also stimulate their brains.

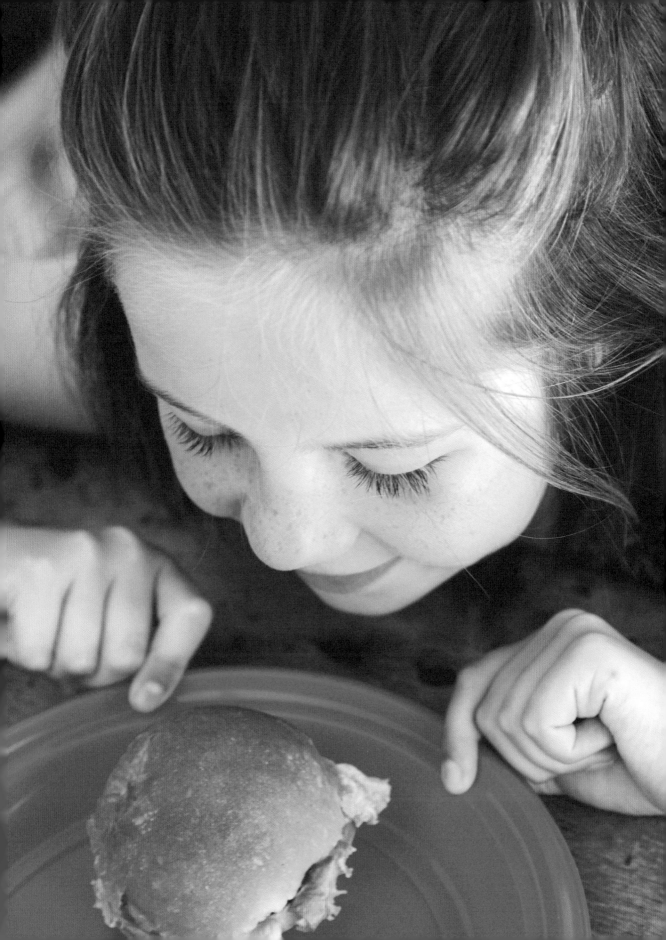

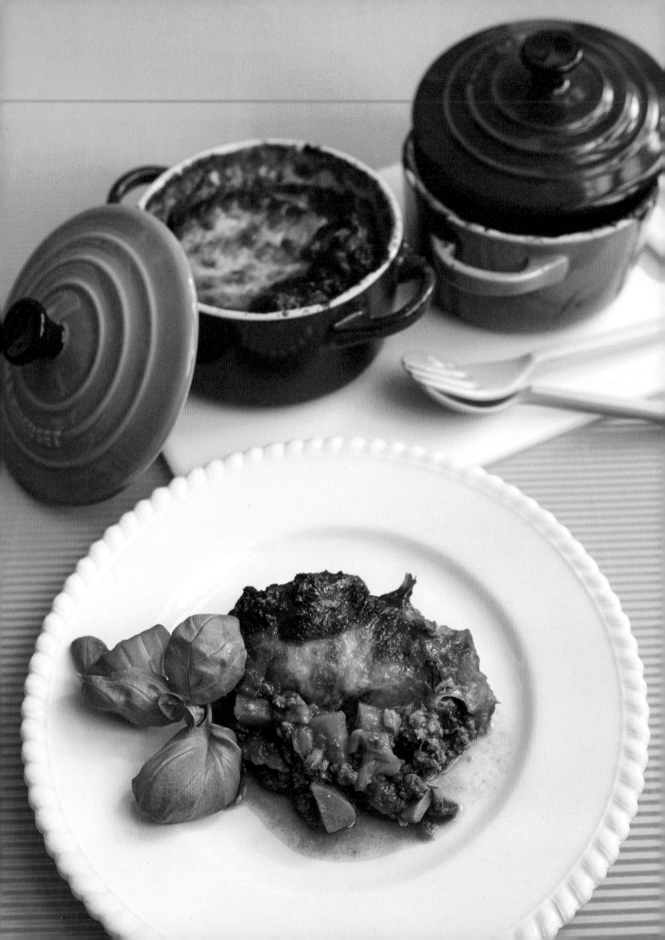

EGGPLANT LASAGNA

This really is a guilt-free, gluten-free pleasure. There is plenty of calcium, protein, and iron in this dish. Don't expect any leftovers!

INGREDIENTS

- 2 medium onions (finely chopped)
- 2 cloves of garlic (finely chopped)
- 2 carrots (finely chopped)
- 1 yellow bell pepper (finely chopped)
- 1 ½ cup / 150 g mushrooms (finely chopped)
- Olive oil
- 2 tsp oregano
- 5 ½ cups / 800 g veal (minced) (omit for vegetarians)
- 2 14 oz / 400 g tins tomatoes (chopped)
- 1 handful of fresh basil (chopped)
- 1 cup / 100 g parmesan (shredded)
- 2 cups / 200 g mozzarella (shredded)
- 3 eggplants (thinly sliced)

PREPARATION

PREHEAT the oven to at 480°F / 250°C.

PLACE a large pan on medium heat with a little bit of olive oil.

ADD the oregano, onions, and garlic and cook for 2 to 3 minutes or until they become translucent.

ADD 1 cup of the chopped vegetables to pan every minute until they are slightly golden.

STIR in the minced veal, breaking it up into little pieces.

Once the veal is cooked, DRAIN any excess fat.

ADD the tomatoes and 1 cup / 240 ml of water.

TURN the heat down to low and let the sauce simmer for an hour with the lid half on.

POUR ¼ of the sauce into a baking dish followed by a layer of thinly sliced eggplant.

SPRINKLE in ⅓ of the mozzarella and parmesan.

REPEAT this process, ending up with a final layer of sauce and a good sprinkle of grated mozzarella and parmesan.

PLACE dish in the oven and bake for 30 to 35 minutes or until the top is crusty and golden.

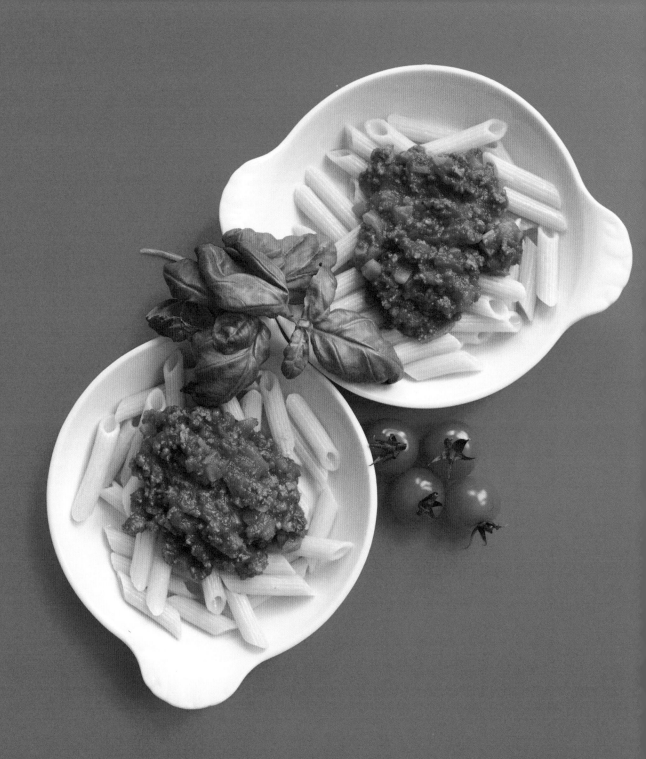

BOLOGNESE

This dish is a favorite of Raphaela (7) and Nathanial (5) who live in Sydney, Australia. Raphaela likes crafts and gymnastics and plays tennis and the piano. When she grows up she wants to be a vet. Nathanial is learning French (just like his sister), builds cities with his Lego, plays soccer, swims on the weekends, and is a pro at judo.

INGREDIENTS

- 2 green bell peppers (finely chopped)
- ¾ cup / 75 g mushrooms (finely chopped)
- ½ medium white onion (chopped into fine pieces)
- 2 ¼ cups / 500 g beef (minced)
- Olive oil
- Vegetable oil
- ⅝ cup / 140 g tomato paste
- 5 cups / 700 g tomato puree
- Rock salt and pepper
- Filtered water
- 1 rosemary sprig
- 2 fresh or dried bay leaves

- Gluten-free pasta

PREPARATION

PLACE the beef into a frying pan with a small amount of vegetable oil and sear until the meat is browned (approximately 8 minutes).

PUT the meat aside and reduce the stove to a medium heat.

ADD 2 tablespoons of olive oil and the chopped vegetables to the pan and brown, stirring regularly until the vegetables are cooked through and slightly caramelized.

ADD some rock salt, then add the meat to the vegetables.

TURN heat to high, then add tomato paste, and stir.

ADD tomato puree and cook for 3 minutes.

LOWER temperature to simmer and stir in 1 ½ cups / 120 ml of water.

ADD one sprig of rosemary and 2 fresh or dried bay leaves.

SIMMER for 25 to 30 minutes, stirring occasionally.

REMOVE bay leaves and rosemary, then serve with gluten-free pasta.

Note: this dishes freezes well for leftovers.

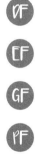

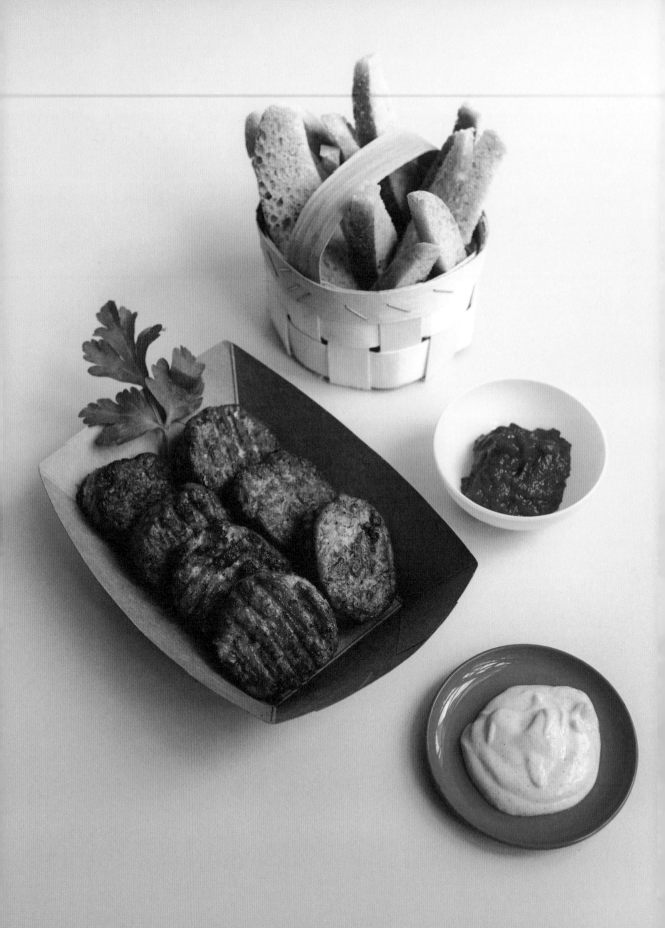

QUINOA & CHICKPEA BURGERS

Filled with protein and whole grains, this is the perfect vegan alternative to a traditional burger.

INGREDIENTS

- ½ cup / 100 g white quinoa
- 1 cup / 240 ml vegetable stock
- 2 cups / 400 g chickpeas (canned or cooked)
- 1 egg
- 1 medium carrot (grated)
- 1 medium zucchini (grated)
- 2 tbsp fresh cilantro (chopped)
- 1 tsp of ground cumin
- Vegetable oil
- Sea salt to taste
- 2 slices of gluten-free bread for breadcrumbs
- Gluten-free bread and salad to serve

PREPARATION

PLACE the vegetable stock and the quinoa in a saucepan and bring to a boil.

COOK for 10 to 15 minutes until the quinoa is soft and all of the liquid has been absorbed. SET aside to cool.

PLACE the gluten-free bread in a blender and mix until a fine powder forms.

ADD the chickpeas, egg, cilantro, zucchini, carrot, and salt into a food processor and blend roughly.

SHAPE the mixture into patties and brush with vegetable oil.

COOK patties in a nonstick frying pan until golden brown (approximately 4 minutes on each side).

SERVE with gluten-free bread and salad.

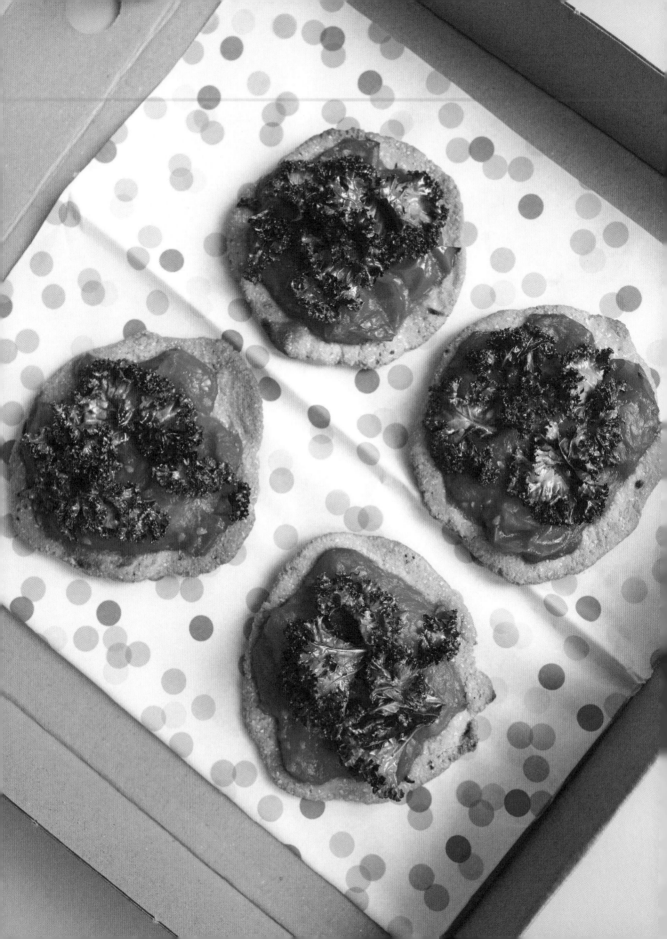

CHICKPEA CRUST PIZZA

Children whose taste buds are conditioned to liking healthy food will delight in this super healthy, guilt-free pizza. It is filled with protein and iron.

INGREDIENTS

Tomato Base Sauce:
- 3 tbsp olive oil
- Salt to taste
- 2 tbsp tomato paste
- 2–3 punnets of cherry tomatoes (halved)

- 2 cups / 185 g chickpea flour
- 1 cup / 240 ml water
- 2 tsp olive oil (for pizza dough)
- 1 pinch salt
- 1 handful of kale (shredded) (substitute with broccoli or basil for fussy eaters)
- 1 tbsp olive oil (for kale)
- ½ cup / 50 g mozzarella or vegan cheese (shredded) (optional)

PREPARATION

PUT cherry tomatoes in a pan on medium heat.

ADD 3 tablespoons of olive oil and salt to taste.

Half COVER the pot so that steam can escape, stirring every few minutes.

After 10 minutes ADD 2 tablespoons of tomato paste.

CONTINUE on medium heat for 25 minutes.

PREHEAT oven to 375°F / 190°C.

LINE a baking sheet with baking paper.

STIR flour, water, olive oil, and salt together in a medium bowl until thoroughly mixed.

SPREAD dough out into a ¼ in / ½ cm circular shape, then bake for 15 to 20 minutes.

MASSAGE kale in small bowl with 1 tablespoon of olive oil.

REMOVE crust from oven and flip upside down on the baking sheet, removing the baking paper.

SPREAD tomato base, then kale, then cheese over the crust.

BAKE for an additional 5 to 7 minutes and serve.

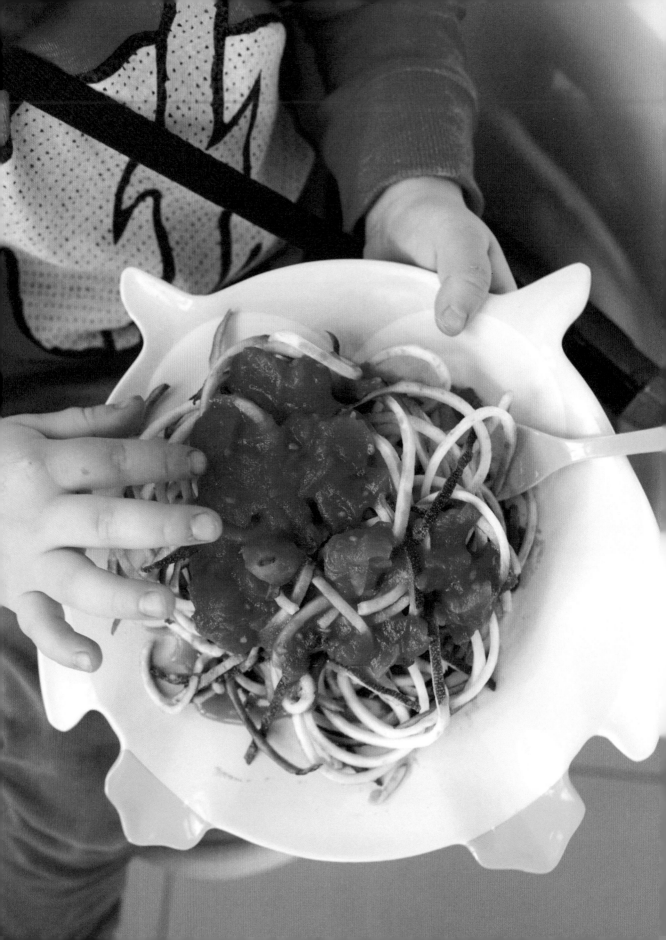

SPIRALIZED ZUCCHINI PASTA

This dish is so easy to make and so healthy! The zucchini is a sneaky and tasty way to get your children to eat their greens.

INGREDIENTS

- 2 large zucchinis (carrots can be added to this for additional color and texture)
- Olive oil
- Fresh basil leaves
- ½ small onion (peeled and chopped into fine pieces)
- ½ garlic clove (crushed)
- 1 cup / 200 g baby tomatoes (chopped)
- 1 scant cup / 200 ml tomato puree
- 1 tbsp tomato paste
- Fresh basil leaves (torn)
- 1 tsp of ricotta
- Parmesan (grated)

PREPARATION

BEGIN by spiralizing the zucchini, then set aside.

HEAT the olive oil in a nonstick pan and sauté the onion, garlic, and baby tomatoes for approximately 7 minutes.

PLACE the onion, tomatoes and garlic in a pot along with the tomato puree, tomato paste, basil, and 1 tablespoon of parmesan.

COVER and SIMMER on a medium heat for approximately 15 minutes, stirring occasionally.

STIR in the ricotta for creaminess and set aside.

ADD 1 tablespoon of olive oil and spiralized zucchini to the nonstick pan for a few moments until it becomes tender.

STIR in the zucchini pasta, then sprinkle parmesan and some fresh basil leaves on top.

If your children are not fussy eaters, try adding olives and pine nuts.

STEAK STRIPS

Let's face it, nothing beats a good steak dinner, and when made into strips, it seems even better. Packed with protein, iron, and B12, this is a dream dinner for a growing child. Remember to get grass-fed organic beef, it is the best!

INGREDIENTS

- 2 7 oz / 200 g steaks (rib-eye or fillet)
- Extra virgin olive oil
- 1 tsp sea salt
- 1 tbsp fresh rosemary (leaves picked)
- ½ tbsp dried oregano
- 1 clove garlic (crushed)
- ½ lemon (juiced)

PREPARATION

BLEND rosemary, oregano, and garlic together, then put mixture in a bowl.

ADD in the extra virgin olive oil and lemon juice, then soak the steaks in the mixture to marinate for at least an hour.

GET a medium sauce pan and heat at high.

PLACE 1 steak at a time and cook each side for 3 minutes, until each side is golden.

Once both steaks are cooked, TURN the heat down to medium and put 2 tablespoons of water in the pan.

ADD a lid and let steaks cook for 5 minutes.

REMOVE the steak and cut into strips.

SERVE with cherry tomatoes and Sweet Potato & Parsnip Fries (see recipe page 124).

FISH PIE

This take on a traditional shepherd's pie is a great dish for smaller children as it's easy to swallow. It is filled with protein, good carbohydrates, omegas, and zinc. Allegra loves this dish and always asks for more!

INGREDIENTS

- 2.2 lb / 1 kg sweet potatoes
- 1 carrot (peeled)
- ¼ cup / 40 g peas
- 1 lemon
- 1 tsp lemon zest shaving
- 2 cups / 600 ml oat cream
- 10.5 oz / 300 g salmon fillets
- 10.5 oz / 300 g haddock fillets
- 4.4 oz / 125 g raw king prawns (peeled)
- Olive oil
- 1 large handful spinach (chopped) (optional)
- ½ medium onion (peeled and thickly sliced)
- 1 bay leaf
- 1 bushy thyme sprig
- 1 tsp shredded lemon zest
- 1 heaping cup / 31 g flat leaf parsley (finely chopped)

PREPARATION

PREHEAT oven to 390°F / 200°C and bring salted water to a boil in a large pot.

PEEL your sweet potatoes and the carrot, CUT them into 3/4 in / 2 cm chunks and set aside.

WASH the spinach thoroughly and set aside.

COOK your potatoes until they are soft.

CUT the salmon and haddock into small chunks and add them to a baking tray with the peeled prawns.

SQUEEZE juice and sprinkle the lemon zest on fish mixture, then drizzle with olive oil and add a pinch of salt and pepper.

ADD the vegetables and stir them into the mixture.

When your potatoes are cooked, DRAIN them in a colander and return them to the pan. DRIZZLE potatoes with some olive oil and add a pinch of salt and pepper.

MASH potatoes until nice and smooth, then spread evenly over the top of the fish and grated vegetables.

PLACE in the oven for about 40 minutes, or until cooked through. SERVE with parsley when crispy and golden on top.

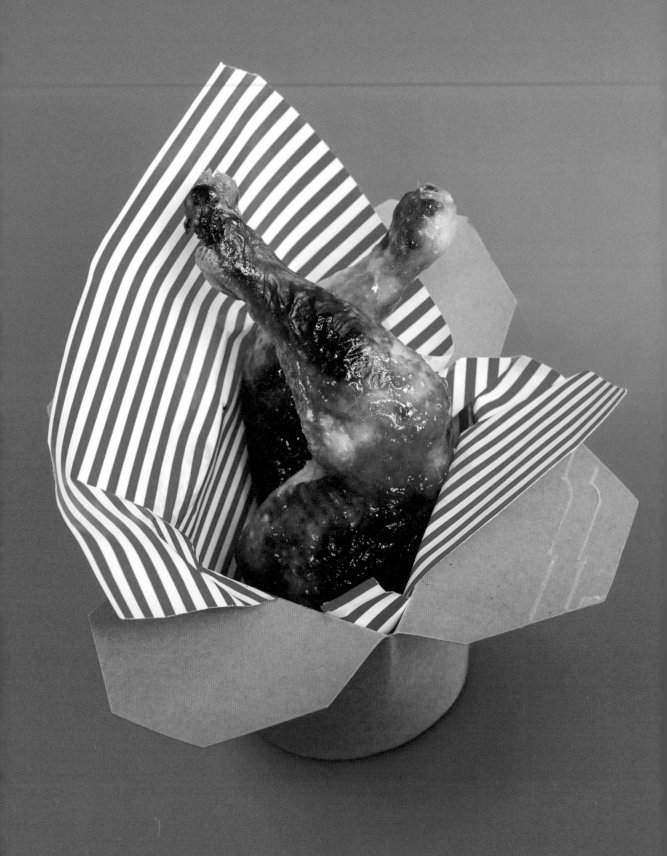

HONEY MUSTARD CHICKEN THIGHS

This is a fun, protein-rich recipe for kid's dinners or parties.

INGREDIENTS

- 6 chicken thighs

Glaze:
- ¾ cup / 225 ml honey
- ½ cup / 125 g prepared mustard
- 1 tbsp cider vinegar

PREPARATION

COMBINE glaze mixture in a bowl with chicken and refrigerate between 1 to 12 hours.

PREHEAT oven to 350°F / 180°C.

BRUSH thighs with glaze and and pop them into the oven for 25 to 30 minutes.

SERVE with Sweet Potato & Parsnip Fries (see recipe page 124).

SIDES

These sides dishes make delicious additions to any meal and are fantastic for sharing at family dinners and children's parties. They also make regular dishes more creative and fun.

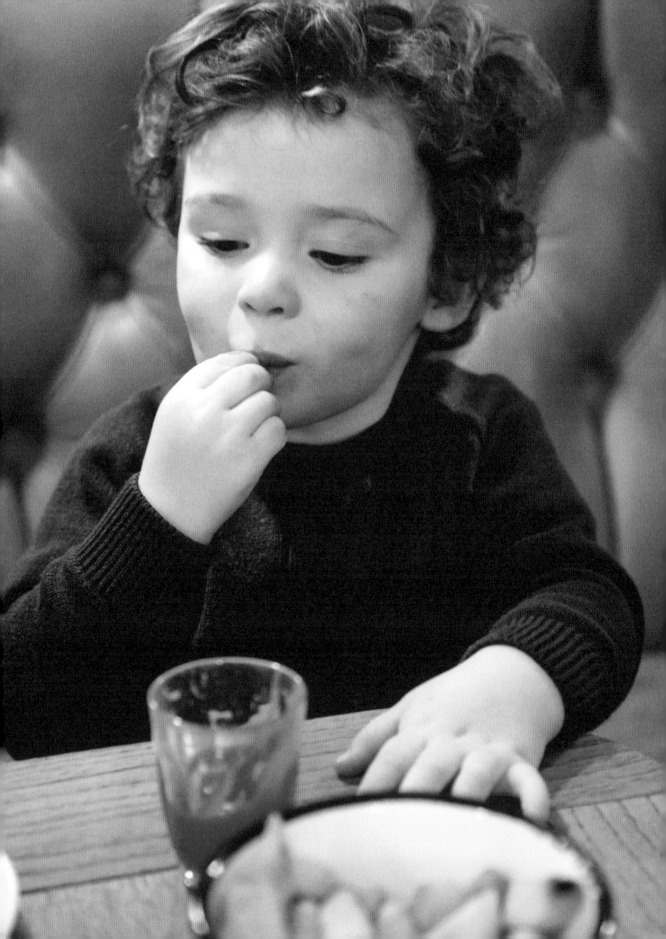

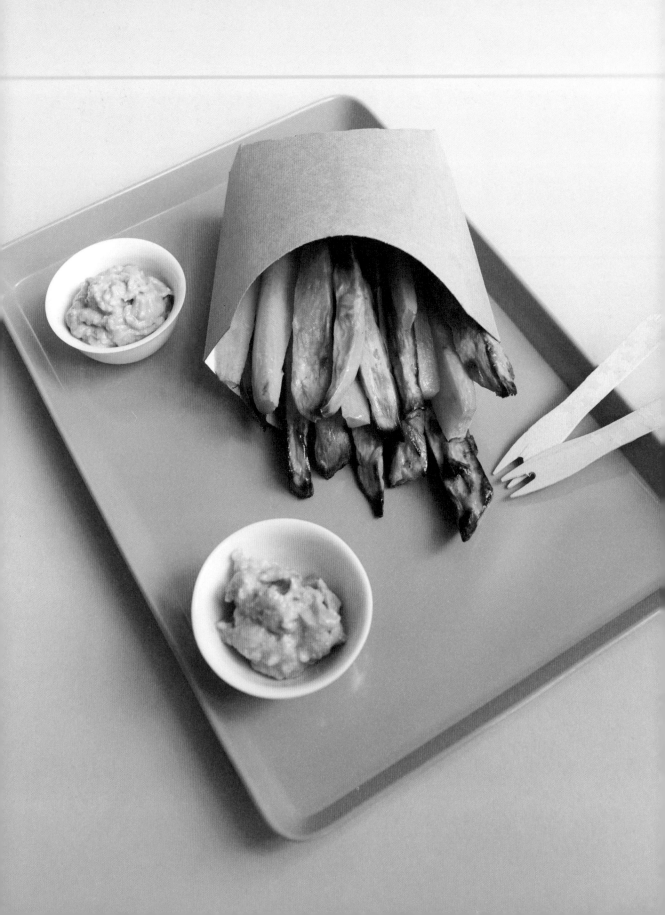

SWEET POTATO & PARSNIP FRIES

Brightly-colored fries, what a surprise! Packed with vitamins A, C, and fiber, you really will be happy when your child asks for more.

INGREDIENTS

- 2.2 lb / 1 kg sweet potato (peeled)
- 1 cup / 500 g parsnips (or carrots) (peeled)
- 2 tsp olive oil
- 2 tsp coconut oil
- 1 tsp sea salt flakes

PREPARATION

PREHEAT oven to 390°F / 200°C.

CUT the sweet potatoes and parsnips into long pieces and place into a bowl, coating them with the oils and salt.

PLACE sweet potatoes and parsnips on a baking tray and bake for 15 minutes.

TURN over (applying extra oil if necessary) and bake for another 10 minutes until fries become crispy.

CAULIFLOWER RICE

Turn cauliflower into rice in this dreamy, creamy dish suddenly packed with the goodness of phyto-chemicals and B12.

INGREDIENTS

- 1 cauliflower
- 1 tbsp olive oil
- 1 zucchini, cut into cubes
- Coconut oil for cooking
- Rock salt to taste

PREPARATION

BREAK apart the cauliflower into large pieces with your hands.

PLACE the cauliflower into a food processor, not filling it to the very top.

PULSE the cauliflower until it is in tiny pieces. If you do not have a food processor, then you can use a grater. The cauliflower granules can be used raw, as it now is, or continue to cook, to make it more like rice.

To cook, WARM a tablespoon of olive oil in a pan on medium heat.

ADD the cauliflower granules and sprinkle with rock salt.

COOK on medium heat for 5 to 8 minutes, until the rice is as tender as you like.

Then ADD a small dollop of coconut oil to a medium size saucepan.

ADD the chopped zucchini to the pan, cooking at medium heat for 5 minutes or until it is soft. Remaining cauliflower rice can be refrigerated or frozen for future use.

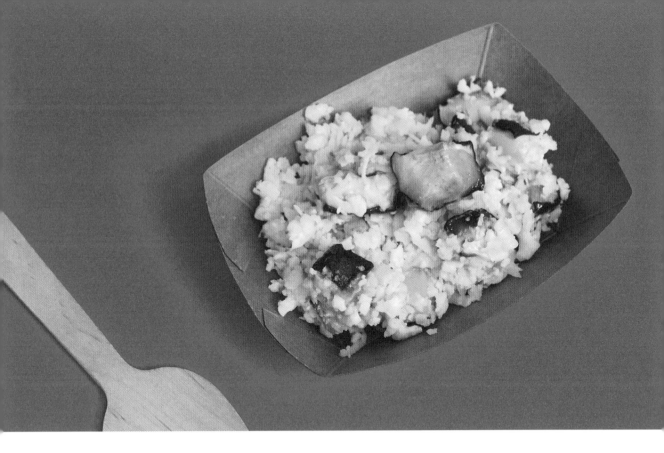

CAULIFLOWER MASH

Kiddies love cauliflower mash, you will find it disappears in seconds. Packed with vitamins B, C, and K, as well as high in antioxidants, you will be happy when your child tries to lick the plate.

INGREDIENTS

- ⅜ cup / 100 ml oat cream
- 1 cauliflower head
- ¼ cup / 60 ml olive oil
- 1 tsp truffle salt

PREPARATION

In a small pot, BRING filtered water to boil with a pinch of salt.

ADD the cauliflower and cook until it becomes soft, then drain the water.

In a large bowl, ADD the cauliflower, oat cream, olive oil, and truffle salt.

USE a blender to blend until a smooth consistency is formed.

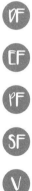

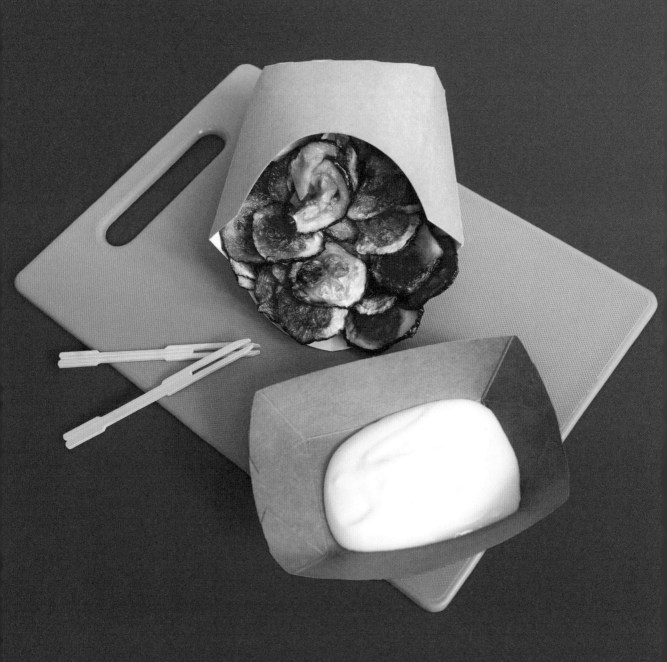

ZUCCHINI CHIPS

Crunchy zucchini chips are an easy way to pack in vitamin C and minerals and they go great with Honey Mustard Chicken Thighs (see recipe page 120).

INGREDIENTS

- 2 large zucchinis (sliced thinly)
- 1 tbsp olive oil
- ½ tbsp Himalayan pink salt

PREPARATION

PREHEAT oven to 320°F / 160°C and line baking trays with baking paper.

PLACE zucchini slices on baking tray.

BRUSH with oil and sprinkle with salt.

BAKE for about 20 minutes, or until crispy and golden.

SWEET CARROTS

Sweet carrots are an easy sell, kids love their sweetness and bright color.
Lucky thing as they are high in carotenoids and great for eyesight.

INGREDIENTS

- 2 lb / 1 kg carrots (chopped and peeled)
- 2 tbsp olive oil
- 1 tsp Maunka honey
- 1 tsp xylitol
- 1 pinch of Himalayan pink salt

PREPARATION

In a medium pot, BOIL water and add a pinch of salt.

ADD the carrots and cook for 5 minutes, or until tender.

Once the carrots are cooked, DRAIN all the water, leaving the carrots in the pot.

SWITCH to low heat and add the olive oil, honey, salt, and xylitol to a pan.

Once the sauce has melted together, MIX it in with the carrots and serve.

PEA PUREE

Sweet pea puree is a tasty side dish that has anti-inflammatory properties and is high in vitamins and minerals. The green color gives it superhero powers and we have created this in honor of our favorite superheroes, Waldorf and Rex, who love playing with trains, racecars, and motorbikes.

INGREDIENTS

- 2 ⅔ cups / 400 g fresh garden peas
- 2 shallots
- 1 tbsp coconut oil
- ½ lemon (juiced)
- ¾ cup / 200 ml Oat Milk (see recipe page 21)

PREPARATION

PLACE peas in a pot of boiling water with a dash of salt.

COOK peas until tender, then run them under cold water for 5 minutes to keep their bright green color.

BLITZ the shallots in a food processor, then cook them in a pan at medium heat with coconut oil until they turn translucent.

PUT cooked shallots, peas, lemon juice, and oat milk in the food processor and blitz for 2 minutes until ultra smooth.

SERVE immediately.

TREATS & SWEETS

Just because we believe in clean eating doesn't mean we want your children to go without indulgences. We have created these delicious, mouthwatering alternatives that are so yummy your kids will never know they are good for them. Please keep in mind that these treats and sweets do have natural sugars and good fats in them, which should be eaten in moderation.

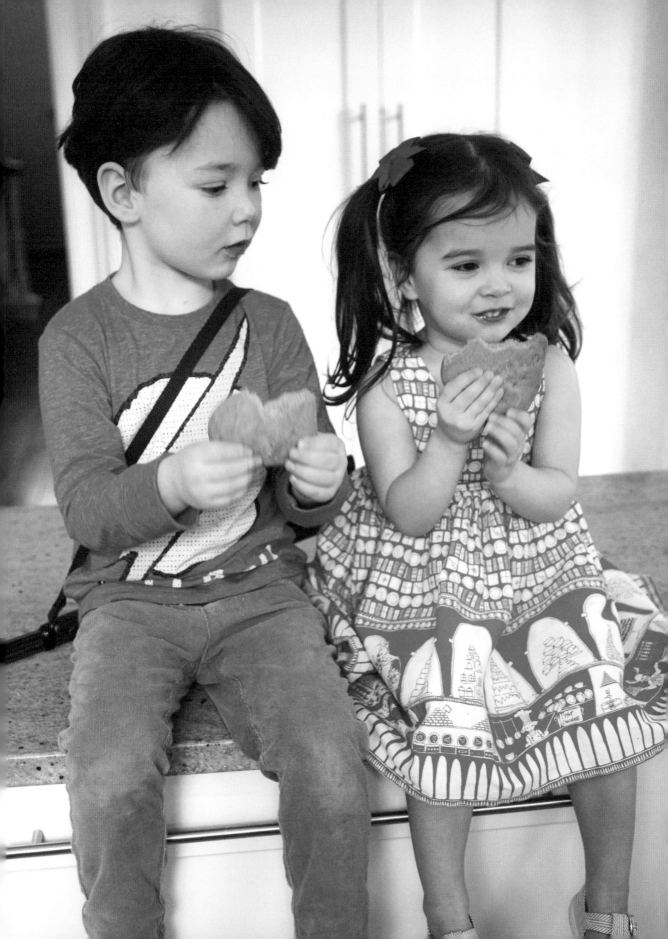

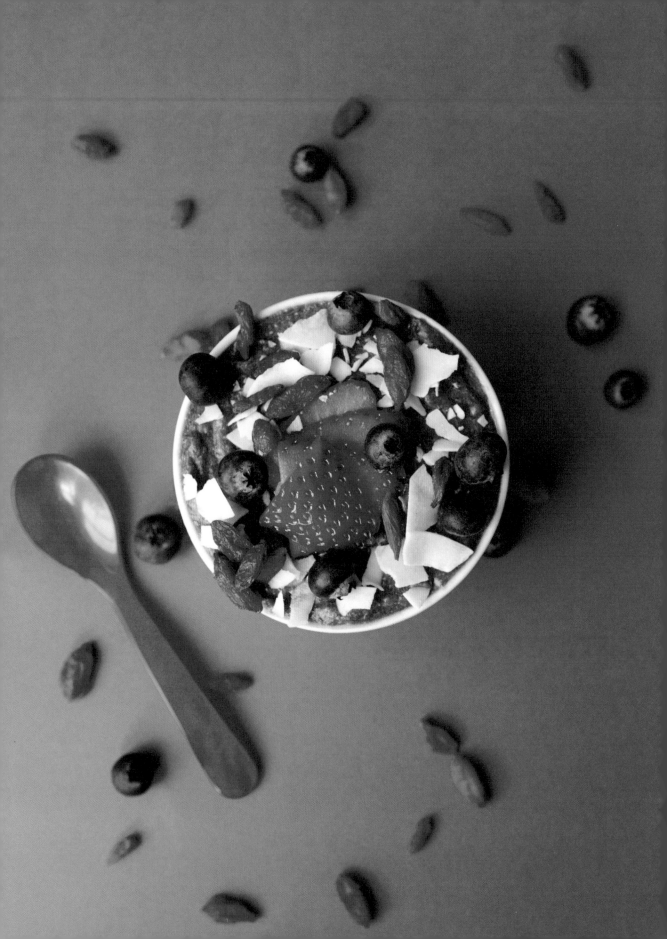

RAW CACAO & AVOCADO MOUSSE

Filled with the goodness of avocado, this mousse brings together good fats, proteins, and potassium. Your children will never know how good it is for them as they devour every bite!

INGREDIENTS

(Serves 4)

- 1 cup / 225 g Medjool dates
- 2 ripe avocados
- 1 small banana
- ¼ cup / 30 g raw cacao powder
- ½ cup / 120 ml milk of your choice (coconut, almond, etc.)

PREPARATION

ADD dates into a food processor and blend until yielding a smooth paste.

ADD remaining ingredients and process until smooth and creamy.

PUT into the fridge to chill for an hour before serving.

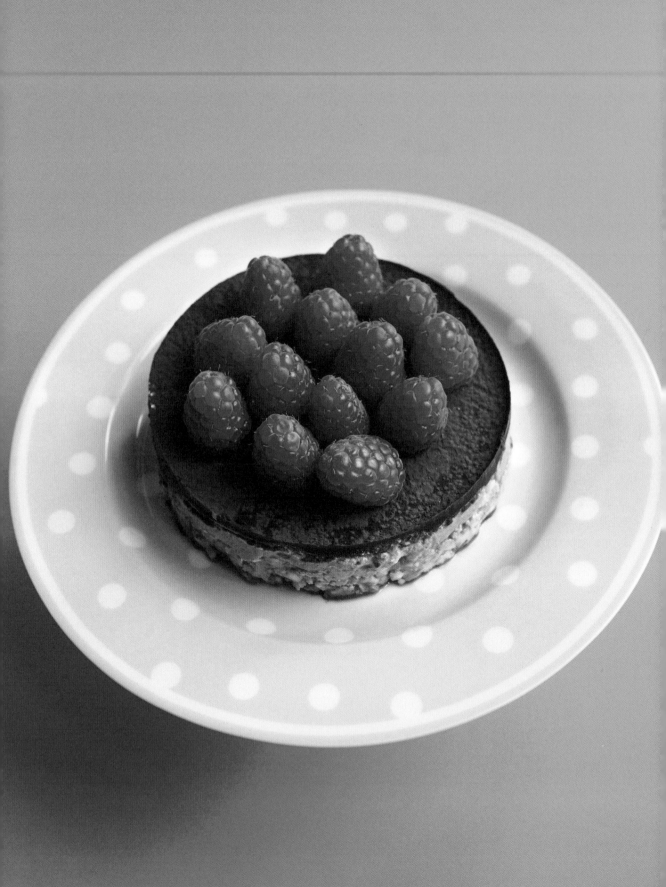

CHOCO PRINCESS LAYER SLICE

This pretty pink cake is made in honor of our favorite princesses, Allegra and Coco. Allegra loves pink and wears a dress better than anyone we know. Coco, seven, is the coolest kid in town, loves to sing and dance and speaks Swedish and English. This dish is also packed with omegas to give you beautiful skin and antioxidants to make you glow and feel good.

INGREDIENTS

Base:
- ½ cup / 50 g walnuts
- ½ cup / 50 g raw cashews
- 2 tbsp coconut oil

Pink Layer:
- ⅓ cup / 80 ml beet juice
- 1 cup / 240 ml coconut milk
- ¼ cup / 60 ml rice malt or maple syrup
- ¾ cup / 70 g desiccated coconut
- ¼ cup / 30 g frozen raspberries
- 1 handful of almonds (sliced)

Choco Top:
- ½ cup / 110 ml coconut oil
- ½ cup / 120 ml maple or rice malt syrup
- 1 cup / 120 g raw cacao

PREPARATION

First BLEND all of the base ingredients until smooth.

LINE a cake tin with baking paper or grease with coconut oil.

POUR base mixture flat into the tin and place in the freezer for at least 20 minutes.

To make the pink layer, BLEND the beet juice, coconut milk, and maple or rice malt syrup until smooth.

ADD the desiccated coconut, half of the raspberries and almonds, and pulse lightly, keeping a chunky consistency.

PLACE this layer on top of the base and refreeze for at least 20 minutes.

For the final layer, HEAT coconut oil until it liquefies.

MIX maple or rice malt syrup, cacao, and coconut oil together.

Once the ingredients have been mixed well, ALLOW to cool and pour over the other layers.

REFREEZE, then garnish with some raspberries.

After 20 minutes, the cake can be cut into slices to serve.

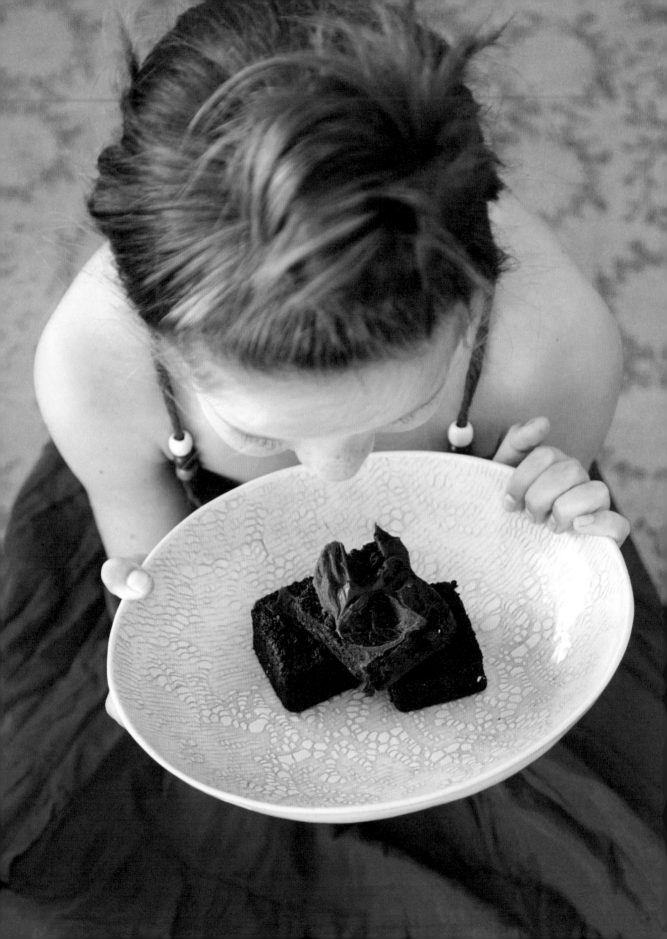

VEGAN CHOCOLATE CAKE

This is a great dish for children who have dairy or egg allergies. Serve at birthday parties or special events so everyone can join in on the fun.

INGREDIENTS

- 2 ½ cups / 315 g all-purpose, gluten-free, self-rising flour
- 1 ½ cups / 320 g xylitol
- 1 cup / 120 g raw cocoa powder
- ½ cup / 85 g raw dairy-free chocolate
- 1 tsp salt
- 2 ⅔ cups / 670 ml coconut milk
- ⅔ cup / 150 ml vegetable oil
- 2 tsp apple cider vinegar
- 1 tsp vanilla extract

Frosting:
- ½ cup / 100 g olive oil margarine
- ½ cup / 95 g vegetable shortening
- 1 ¼ cup / 160 g FTF Icing "Sugar" (see recipe page 160)
- ¼ cup / 30 g raw cocoa powder
- 1 tsp vanilla extract
- 2 tbsp oat cream

PREPARATION

PREHEAT oven to 350°F / 180°C.

GREASE a pair of 8 in / 20 cm round baking pans with coconut oil, then place a circle of parchment paper into the bottom of each pan.

WHISK together the dry ingredients in a large bowl and all of the wet ingredients in another.

POUR both sets of ingredients into a large bowl and mix until combined. Avoid over mixing.

POUR cake mix into both pans and bake in the oven for 40 minutes, or until cooked.

SET the cakes aside to cool completely and make the frosting.

BLEND all the frosting ingredients together (except for the oat cream) until consistency is creamy and can form whipped peaks.

ADD oat cream if you need to make the frosting creamier.

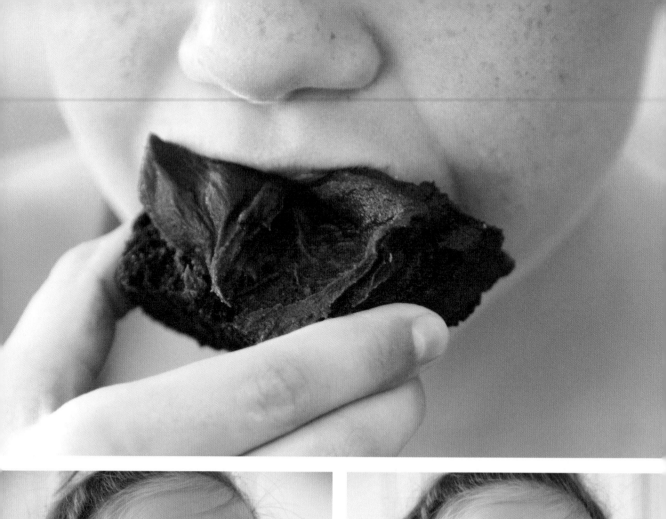
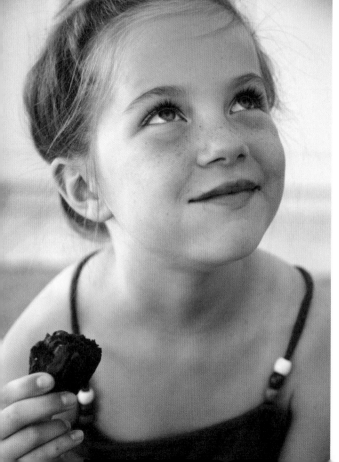
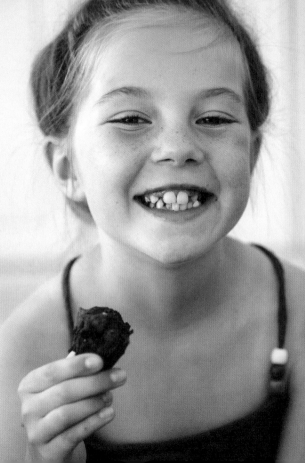

VEGAN CHOCOLATE CAKE

PREPARATION

Once the cakes are both cool, RUN a knife
around the edges of the cake pans.

FLIP the pans over to remove the cakes
and discard the paper lining.

PLACE one of the cakes on top of a cake platter
and frost completely.

PLACE the second cake on top of the frosted one
and cover with remaining frosting.

STORE cake in a cool place until you're ready to serve.

*Tip: You can test if your cakes are perfectly cooked
by using a simple toothpick trick. Insert a toothpick into
the center of the cake, and if it comes out clean when
you remove it, the cake is done baking.*

FTF SHORTBREAD PASTRY

This delicious pastry is great for pies—we recommend making a few batches and keeping them in the freezer to use when needed.

INGREDIENTS

- 1 ⅔ cups / 225 g gluten-free flour
- 1 pinch salt
- ¼ tsp xanthan gum (optional, but holds the mixture together well)
- ½ cup / 112 g coconut oil
- ¼ cup / 56 g coconut sugar or xylitol
- 1 egg yolk
- 2 tbsp cold filtered water

PREPARATION

SIFT the flour, salt, and xanthan gum in a large bowl.

RUB the coconut oil into the flour until it forms a breadcrumb-like consistency.

STIR in the coconut sugar or xylitol and egg yolk.

ADD a small amount of water to make a dough.

WRAP the dough in clear wrap and put in the fridge to set for approximately 20 minutes.

CHOCOLATE SHORTBREAD COOKIES

These chocolate shortbread cookies are filled with the taste of naughtiness but the sweetness of FTF goodness. They're loaded with chia seeds and flaxseeds, which together make a dream team. The combo is high in fiber, antioxidants, and omega-3 fatty acids, not to mention magnesium and phosphorous to promote healthy bones. Who knew healthy cookies could be so good for you? We haven't even covered all of the goodness yet. These cookies call for flavonoid-filled raw chocolate that also boast B vitamins. Flavonoids are known for their anti-inflammatory benefits, cardiovascular benefits, anti-stress properties.

INGREDIENTS

(Makes 12 Cookies)

- 11.5 oz / 325 g FTF Short-bread Pastry (see recipe page 142)
- ½ cup / 90 g raw chocolate
- 3 tbs chia flaxseed powder
- 1 tube of decorating icing
- 12 dried blackberries or cherries

PREPARATION

PREHEAT the oven to 350°F / 180°C.
MAKE sure the pastry is at room temperature before you begin.
PLACE the raw chocolate in a small saucepan and cook on low for 3 to 5 minutes.
MAKE sure you heat the chocolate until it is soft (do not completely melt the chocolate otherwise it will burn).
KNEAD the softened chocolate through the pastry until it is completely brown (not marbled).
ADD the chia and flaxseed powder then knead until it is completely mixed through.
PLACE the dough in the freezer for 20 minutes.
Once the dough has hardened, SPRINKLE some flour on the table and on a rolling pin, then flatten the dough.
Using a star-shaped cookie cutter, CUT out 12 cookies.
ARRANGE cookie dough onto a tray lined with baking paper and place in the oven for 5 to 10 minutes.
Once the cookies have cooled down, USE the decorating icing to make a round mound in the middle of the cookie.
SET dried fruit atop the icing and enjoy!

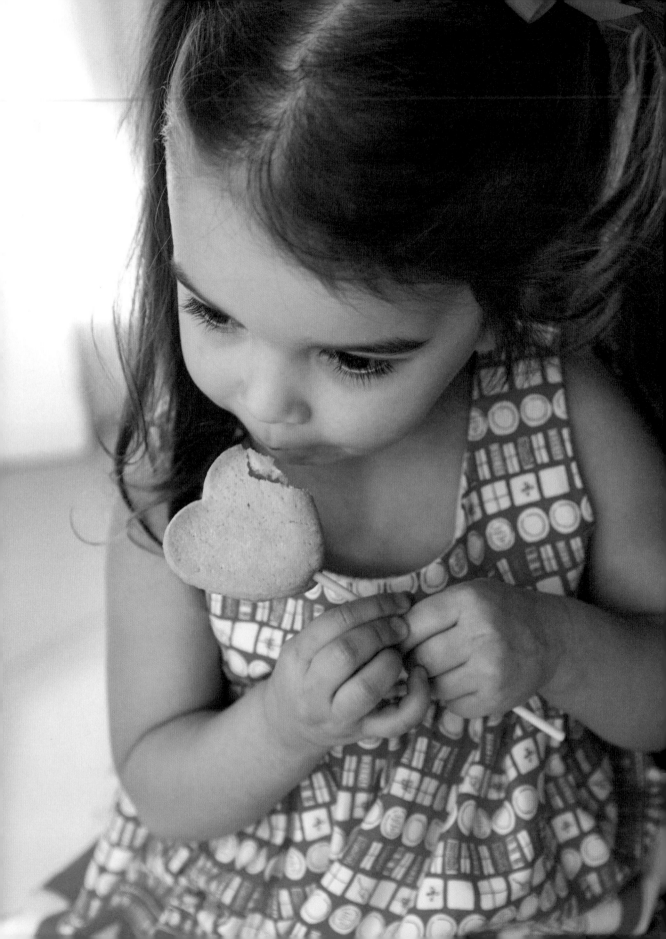

FAIRY WAND SHORTBREAD COOKIES

Children love treats on a stick and these fairy wand biscuits are no different. They are delicious on their own or you can always spread a bit of Un-Nutella (see recipe page 36) on them!

INGREDIENTS

- Coconut oil (melted, to grease)
- 1 cup / 250 g coconut oil
- ½ cup / 120 ml maple syrup
- 2 cups / 300 g gluten-free plain flour (sifted)
- ½ cup / 90 g rice flour (sifted)
- FTF Raw Berry Jam (see recipe page 160)

PREPARATION

PREHEAT oven to 300°F / 150°C.

BRUSH 2 baking trays with melted coconut oil to grease.

USE a hand mixer to beat the coconut oil and maple syrup together in a bowl until creamy.

MIX both flours.

ADD the combined flour slowly, beating on low speed until almost fully combined.

MIX the dough together in a bowl with your hands, then knead on a lightly floured surface.

FLATTEN dough with a rolling pin before cutting out stars or hearts with a cookie cutter.

BAKE the shortbread for approximately 15 minutes or until golden brown.

KEEP shortbread on trays and set aside to cool for 10 minutes, then transfer them to a wire rack to cool completely.

To finish your fairy wands, COAT 2 shortbread cookies of the same shape with FTF raw berry jam, then press together with a popsicle stick in between.

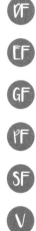

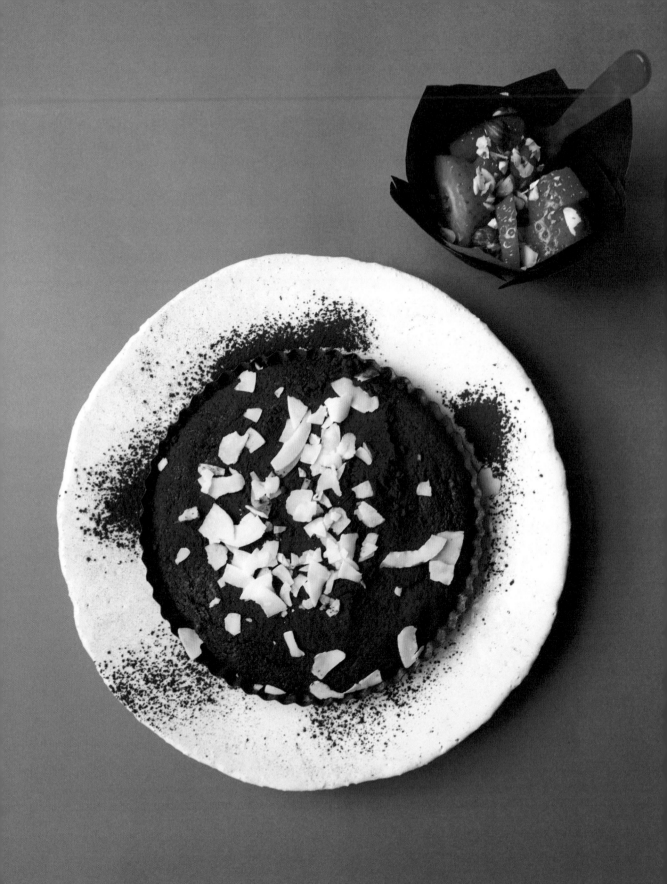

CACAO BEET BROWNIES

This healthy and delicious take on traditional brownie sneaks in beets, which are high in antioxidants, iron, magnesium, and potassium. They're also a great source of folic acid.

INGREDIENTS

- 4 large beets
- 2 tsp vanilla extract
- 3 eggs
- ¼ cup / 50 g coconut sugar
- ¾ cup / 90 g raw cacao powder
- ½ cup / 100 ml coconut oil (melted)
- 1 tsp gluten-free baking powder
- ½ cup / 50 g almond meal
- ⅓ cup / 50 g chopped dates

PREPARATION

PREHEAT oven to 350°F / 180°C.

BRING the beets to a boil in a pan of water (with a pinch of salt) for 45 to 60 minutes, or until tender.

DRAIN water and set beets aside to cool.

Wearing gloves, PEEL away the outer beet skin.

CHOP the beets into cubes and blend in a food processor until they become a paste.

SQUEEZE the paste through a sieve into a bowl.

With an hand mixer, BEAT the vanilla extract, eggs, and coconut sugar until fluffy.

FOLD in the cacao, coconut oil, baking powder, almond meal, and dates.

POUR into baking tins and bake for 25 minutes (the brownies should still be slightly gooey in the middle).

SET brownies aside to cool before cutting them.

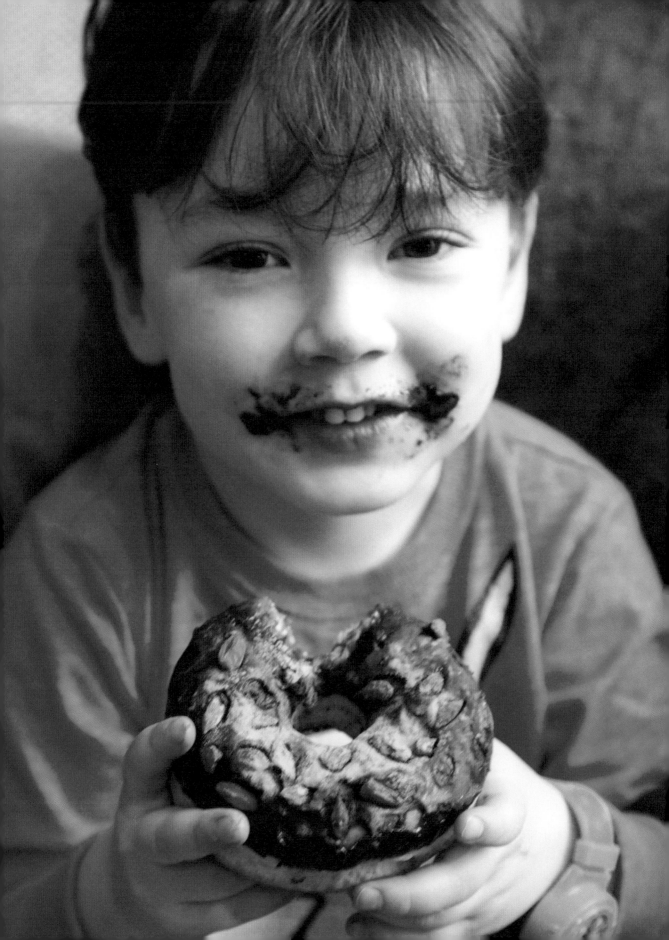

BAKED DOUGHNUTS

Kids fight over these scrumptious doughnuts, they are so moist and delicious! Play with nuts, berries, seeds, and superfood powders to create creative and different garnishes each time.

INGREDIENTS

Doughnuts:
- 1 ½ cup / 145 g almond meal
- ¼ cup / 50 g coconut sugar
- ¼ tsp salt
- ¼ tsp nutmeg
- 1 egg (whisked)
- ½ tsp cinnamon
- ½ tsp baking soda
- 1 cup / 300 g ripe banana (mashed)
- ¼ cup / 60 ml regular or coconut milk
- 2 tbsp maple syrup
- ½ tsp vanilla bean paste

Raw Choc-Nut Icing:
- 1 cup / 240 g hazelnuts
- ⅓ cup / 80 ml coconut milk
- 1 tsp vanilla bean paste
- ¼ cup / 60 ml maple syrup
- 2 tbsp raw cacao powder

- Dried berries or pistachio powder for garnish

PREPARATION

PREHEAT oven to 350°F / 180°C.

ADD coconut sugar, salt, nutmeg, almond meal, baking soda, and cinnamon to a large bowl.

In a separate bowl, COMBINE banana, egg, coconut milk, vanilla bean paste, and maple syrup.

Gently FOLD these ingredients into the first bowl.

POUR mixture into doughnut tins. If you do not have doughnut tins, use a flat baking tray greased or lined with baking paper. TAKE a small amount of dough and roll a cylinder with your hands. JOIN the ends to make a doughnut shape.

BAKE for 12 minutes, then let doughnuts rest on a cooling rack before frosting.

For the icing RESET oven temperature to 320°F / 160°C.

ROAST hazelnuts for 10 to 12 minutes. Allow hazelnuts to cool before RUBBING OFF their skins.

BLEND hazelnuts in a food processor to create a nut butter. ADD remaining ingredients and blend until fully combined.

USE a butter knife to carefully frost each doughnut with the icing. GARNISH with pistachio powder or dried berries.

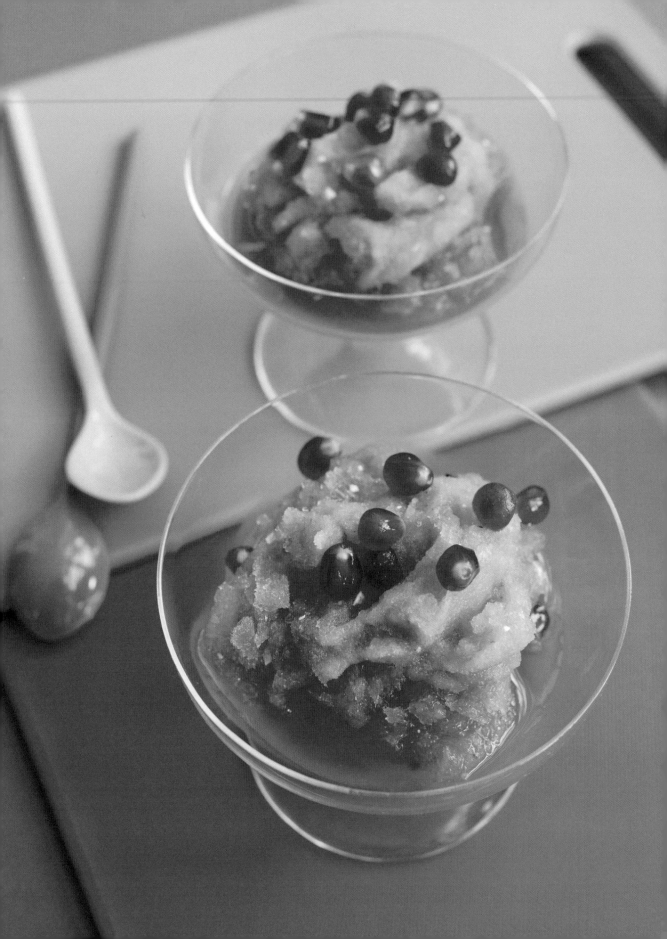

WATERMELON GRANITA

Refreshing and hydrating, this granita will keep kids cool on a hot summer's eve.

INGREDIENTS

- 4 cups / 610 g seedless watermelon (chopped)
- ¼ cup / 60 ml maple syrup
- ¾ cup / 170 ml filtered water
- 1 tbsp lemon juice

PREPARATION

PLACE filtered water and maple syrup into a pot and bring to boil, then add lemon juice.

After a few minutes, TAKE the syrup off the stove and allow to cool.

PLACE the watermelon into a food processor and blend until smooth.

ADD the cooled syrup to the watermelon, then place the mixture in a flat tin.

ALLOW mixture to sit in the freezer for approximately 2 hours.

After the mixture has set, STIR with a fork to break it up into icy shards.

REFREEZE and serve.

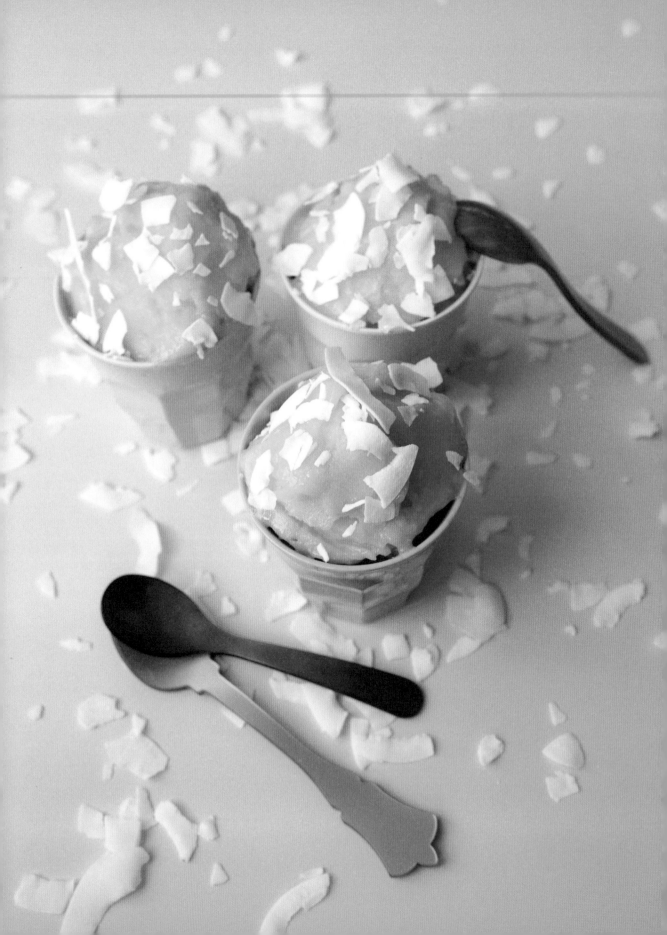

MANGO SORBET

This dairy-free delight is a great alternative to traditional ice cream.

INGREDIENTS

- 6 medium mangoes
  (peeled and sliced)
- 1 egg white
- ½ cup / 120 ml maple syrup
- 1 tsp lemon juice
- 1 cup / 250 ml filtered
  water

PREPARATION

BRING filtered water, maple syrup, and lemon juice to a boil over medium heat.

REMOVE from heat once it's slightly thickened and allow to cool.

In a blender, PUREE the mangoes then add maple syrup and egg white.

FREEZE the mixture until it is semi-frozen.

TAKE mixture out of the freezer and blend until smooth to create a light and fluffy consistency.

REFREEZE until ready to enjoy.

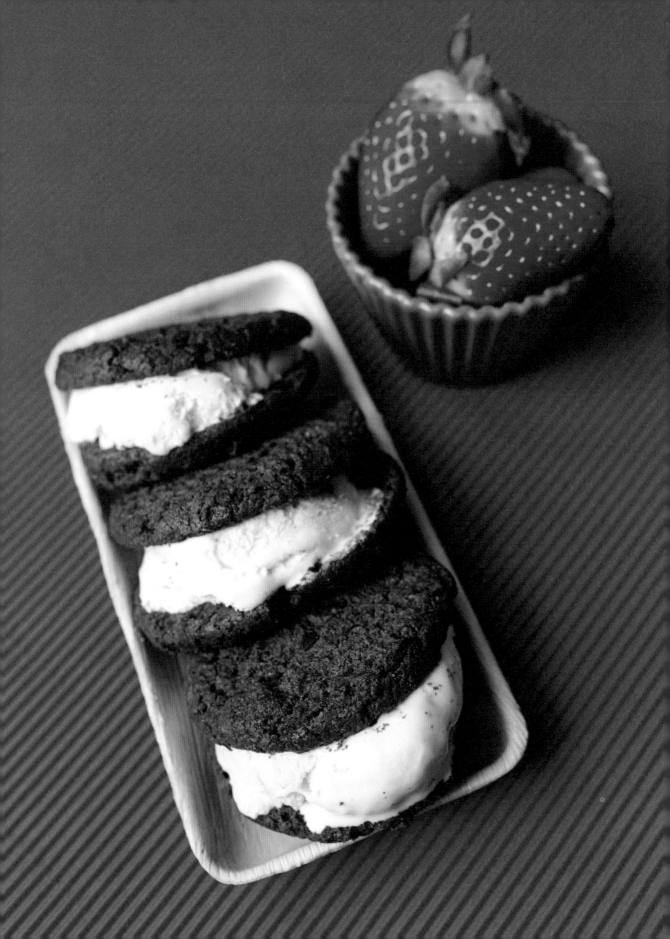

NICE CREAM COOKIE SANDWICH

Yummy scrummy in my tummy! These nice cream sandwiches are a great summer treat.

INGREDIENTS

Nice Cream Center:

- 1 cup / 225 g ripe banana and avocado (sliced)
- 1 cup / 245 g coconut yogurt
- 2 cups / 590 ml coconut cream
- ¾ cup / 180 ml rice malt or maple syrup

Cookies:

- ½ cup / 50 g lightly roasted hazelnuts
- ¼ cup / 20 g desiccated coconut
- 2 tbsp flax meal
- ⅓ cup / 30 g rolled gluten-free oats
- ¾ cup / 115 g sultanas
- ⅓ cup / 75 g Medjool dates
- 2 tsp cinnamon
- 1 tbsp coconut oil (melted)
- 1 tbsp maple syrup
- 1 tsp vanilla bean paste

PREPARATION

Nice Cream Center:

MASH banana and avocado.

COMBINE all ingredients in a bowl, then place the mixture in a zip-close bag.

PLACE bag in the freezer and let sit for 2 to 4 hours.

Once the mixture is frozen, PLACE it in a blender and mix until smooth, then refreeze.

Cookies:

PREHEAT oven to 210°F / 100°C.

PUT all ingredients into your food processor and blend until mixture is sticky when pressed between your fingers.

LINE a tray with baking paper and press 2 tablespoons of your cookie mixture into cookie cutters. You should have enough dough for 12 cookies.

COOK in the oven for approximately 15 minutes, then let cool on a cooling rack. Cookies will slightly harden, but still remain soft and chewy.

LAYER nice cream between two cookies, then refreeze in an airtight container.

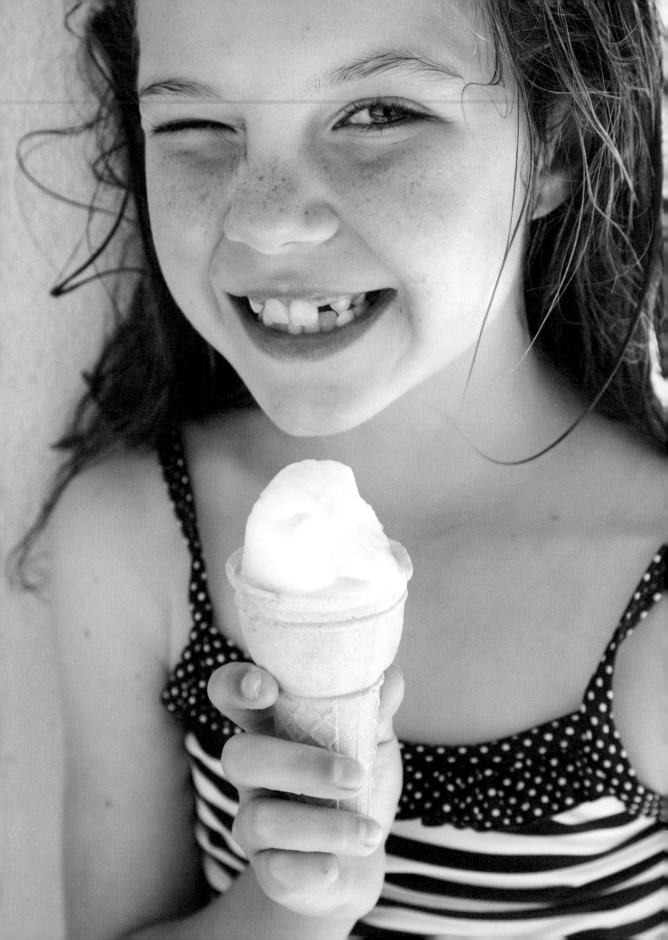

BANANA ICE CREAM

It is super easy to make this creamy banana ice cream and your children won't even know it's dairy free!

INGREDIENTS

- 4 bananas
- 1 tsp vanilla extract
- ½ cup / 120 ml maple syrup
- ½ cup / 150 ml coconut cream
- Raw dark chocolate chunks to taste

PREPARATION

BLEND together bananas, vanilla extract, maple syrup, and coconut cream.

PUT in the freezer for 4 hours.

GARNISH with chocolate chunks and serve.

CONDIMENTS

*We believe that fresh produce is the best produce.
To get the most nutrients out of the food we eat and
give our families, we need to cook with the freshest food
possible. To make sure there are no preservatives or
sneaky additives in our food, it is important to make
our own condiments when possible. This includes our
own nut milks, sauces, and spreads. Most can be
refrigerated and stored, or make great gifts
when visiting friends.*

FTF PEANUT BUTTER

This delicious, nutritious snack is filling and a fun, playful snack for kids of all ages. It's quick and easy to make and they will love it! Spread your FTF homemade peanut butter onto unsalted rice cakes. The peanut butter is filled with protein, vitamin E and magnesium, and the banana and blueberries add natural sweetness. There are plenty of minerals and vitamins in both. Bananas contain a high amount of potassium and vitamin C. While the blueberries are packed with fiber, anti-oxidants, and B6.

INGREDIENTS

- 2 cups / 300 g unsalted peanuts
- Sea salt to taste

PREPARATION

PREHEAT oven to 350°F / 180°C.

PLACE peanuts on a lined baking tray and roast for approximately 10 to 12 minutes. Be careful not to burn them!

LET the peanuts cool completely.

In a food processor, BLEND peanuts until they become a nut butter.

SPRINKLE with some sea salt.

FTF RAW BERRY JAM

INGREDIENTS

- ¼ cup / 60 ml coconut water
- ½ cup / 85 g dates (pitted)
- 2 cups / 320 g raspberries
- Natural sweetener to taste (coconut nectar or maple syrup)
- 2 tbsp chia seeds

Note: When sealed in a jar, this jam will keep in the fridge for four days.

PREPARATION

CHOP dates into fine pieces.

POUR the coconut water into your blender, then add the dates.

BLEND on high for 30 to 60 seconds until the dates have all broken up.

ADD the chia seeds and half of the raspberries, then pulse to break up the berries.

ADD the rest of the raspberries, then pulse on low until achieving a chunky consistency.

If you find the jam tart, MIX in some natural sweetener as desired.

REFRIGERATE for 30 minutes to let chia seeds expand.

FTF ICING "SUGAR"

INGREDIENTS

- 1 ½ cups / 320 g xylitol (granulated)
- 1 tbsp arrowroot

PREPARATION

PLACE the sweetener and arrowroot into your blender.

BLITZ on high until the mixture achieves a smooth, powdered consistency.

KEEP the lid on the blender until the powder settles, then sift to make sure there are no lumps.

FTF ALMOND BUTTER

INGREDIENTS

- 3 cups / 450 g raw almonds
- Filtered water

Note: Almonds can be substituted for any nut of your choice

PREPARATION

SOAK the almonds in filtered water overnight.

The following day, DRAIN and RINSE the almonds.

PREHEAT the oven to 350°F / 180°C.

PLACE the almonds on a baking tray and warm for 5 minutes.

PLACE the almonds in a blender and mix while continuing to scrape down sides of the bowl until they form a smooth texture. (Depending on the strength of your blender, this could take anywhere from 5 to 20 minutes.)

LEAVE raw, add salt to taste, or try blending in something sweet like raw cacao, cinnamon, honey, or desiccated coconut.

FTF MAYONNAISE

INGREDIENTS

- 3 tbsp lemon juice
- 2 tbsp live apple cider vinegar
- 1 ½ tsp mustard (ground)
- 2 tbsp raw honey (or other natural sweetener)
- 1 ¼ tsp Himalayan pink salt
- ½ cup / 110 ml cold-pressed extra virgin olive oil
- ½ cup / 110 g solid coconut oil

PREPARATION

In a food processor, BLEND lemon juice, honey, vinegar, mustard, and salt.

While food processor is still mixing, slowly ADD in the olive oil.

Next ADD in the in coconut oil and continue mixing until smooth.

Once the mixture reaches a creamy consistency, POUR it into a serving bowl or sealable container.

USE immediately or store in the fridge for up to a week.

NUTRIENT FACTS

Vitamin A (Retinol)
Vitamin A is needed for vision, skin structure, and proper functioning of our mucous membranes, digestive system, and lungs. This vitamin plays a role in bone growth and normal development, so it's especially important in our younger years. It is also an antioxidant that boosts our immune system and promotes detoxification.

Vitamin B1 (Thiamine)
Vitamin B1 is needed to release energy from carbohydrates as it converts blood sugar into energy. It is also involved in the normal functioning of the nervous system, brain, heart, and digestive system. Vitamin B1 is also needed to produce red blood cells and promote a healthy immune system.

Vitamin B2 (Riboflavin)
Vitamin B2 is essential for growth and development. It plays a role in tissue respiration and the synthesis of steroids, red blood cells, and glycogen (a form or glucose). It also helps to maintain healthy mucous membranes, skin, eyes, and nervous systems. Four other important roles of vitamin B2 include energy metabolism, drug metabolism, lipid metabolism, and antioxidant protection. It also activates folate and B6.

Vitamin B3 (Niacin)
Vitamin B3 is needed to release energy from food, maintain healthy skin mucous membranes, and promote a fully functioning nervous system. It also helps keep your digestive system strong and blood sugar regulated. In addition, it also metabolizes fats, proteins, and carbohydrates.

Vitamin B5 (Pantothenic Acid)
Vitamin B5 is essential for life. It turns food (carbs) into energy (glucose) and has a central role in the metabolism of fatty acids and protein. It improves the body's resistance to stress and strengthens the immune system with its antibody production.

Vitamin B6 (Pyridoxine)
Vitamin B6 helps produce red bloods cells in the body, metabolize carbohydrates and fats, and improve oxygenation of tissues. It also supports transmitters in the brain and nervous system.

Vitamin B9 (Folate – Folic acid)
Vitamin B9 is essential for cell growth and metabolism. Folate is a natural source of B9 found in food while folic acid is man-made and added to food. Vitamin B9 is one of the most crucial nutrients for your body as it plays an important role in DNA synthesis and repair. It famously helps with the development of healthy babies, lowering cancer risks, maintaining healthy organs, providing neurological support, and promoting digestive health. These B vitamins are cliquey and like to work together in synergy!

Vitamin B12 (Cobalamin)
Vitamin B12 is required for normal cell division, as well as blood formation and function. It maintains normal bone marrow and also helps process folic acid. It's needed for energy production throughout the body.

Vitamin C (Ascorbic Acid)
Vitamin C is involved in the production of collagen, the protein in connective tissue. Vitamin C helps ensure normal structure and function of blood vessels and connective tissues such as skin, cartilage, and bone, making it a player in the body's healing process. Vitamin C also supports healthy neurological function and contributes to the absorption of iron in plant foods. With its antioxidant activities, vitamin C can help protect cells from free radicals. Vitamin C even boasts antihistamine properties.

Vitamin D (Calcitirol)
Vitamin D is made from ultra violet rays on the skin and can be found in food, although few ingredients contain significant amounts. Our bodies convert the vitamin in the liver and the kidney so it can help with the process of cell division, controlling phosphorous, and normal bone mineralization.

Vitamin E (Tocopherol)

Vitamin E is a group of compounds called tocopherols. Alpha tocopherol is the most active of the group and acts as an antioxidant. It's required to protect cells against damage by free radicals like the oxidation of lipids in the cell membranes. We love it because it is an intracellular antioxidant that improves blood flow and reduces cognitive decline.

Vitamin K

Vitamin K is essential for the clotting of blood and is also required for normal bone structure. It has an anti-inflammatory effect which helps prevent excessive bone loss and maintain bone mass because it's used to activate osteocalcin, the major non-collagenous protein in bone.

Essential Fatty Acids

EFA's are vital poly-unsaturated fats for the human body. These fats are needed for normal growth and development for children of all ages. Linoleic acid is the principal precursor of omega-6 fatty acids. Omega-6 play a crucial role in pro-inflammatory reactions, such as blood clots, allergic reactions, healthy skin, and they can help combat against bacteria and viruses. Linolenic acid/alpha-linolenic acid (ALA) is the precursor for omega-3 fatty acids. These fats are an important component of nerve cell membranes, helping the nerves communicate with each other and maintain a healthy brain. Omega-3 fats also have an anti-inflammatory effect on joints and can help with muscle stiffness. They even help blood sugar and cholesterol levels, keeping us fit!

Calcium

Calcium is needed for healthy bones and teeth. Calcium also plays an essential role in intracellular signaling and is therefore necessary for nerve and muscle function. It is also involved in blood clotting. Calcium intake is important for achieving peak bone mass early in life to try and fight against the rate of age-related bone loss as we get older.

Chromium

Chromium is an essential mineral required by the body in trace amounts. This mineral is an active component of glucose tolerance factor (GTF) and plays a fundamental role in controlling blood sugar levels. The primary function of GTF is to increase the action of insulin. Insulin is the hormone responsible for carrying sugar (glucose) into the cells where it can be used for energy.

Iron

Iron is required for the formation of hemoglobin in red blood cells. Hemoglobin transports oxygen around the body. It is also required for normal energy and metabolism, as well as the metabolism of drugs and foreign substances that need to be removed from body. The immune system also requires iron to function properly.

Magnesium

Magnesium is present in all tissues, including bone. It is required for normal metabolism and electrolyte balance. It is also needed for muscle function and tooth structure.

Phosphorus

Phosphorus is present in all plant and animal cells. Our skeletons house 80% of the body's phosphorous as calcium salts. Phosphorous is essential for bone and tooth structure, and is also a component of DNA and RNA.

Potassium

Potassium is found in body fluids and is essential for water and electrolyte balance. It supports the proper functioning of cells, including nerves, and preserves bone density. Potassium can even have a beneficial effect on people with high blood pressure.

Zinc

Zinc is present in many enzymes and is crucial for cell division making it essential for growth and tissue repair. It is also necessary for normal reproductive development. Zinc boosts the immune system and supports wound healing.

FOOD STORES

ASIA PACIFIC

AUSTRALIA
Adelaide
- Goodies & Grains
- Healthy Life
- Natural Food Barn
- Romeo's Organic Wholefoods

Brisbane
- Fundies Wholefood Market
- The Green Edge
- Vive Health
- Vitality Health Foods
- Wray Organic

Melbourne
- Aunt Maggies
- Botanical Cuisine
- David Jones Foodhall
- Friends of the Earth Co-op
- Great Earth
- Joe's Organic Market
- Kew Organics
- The Little Hen
- Miss Spelts Grains & Goodies
- Prahran Health Foods
- Spelt Quinoa
- TOFWD* The Organic Food and Wine Deli
- Terra Madre
- Wholefoods Food Store

Perth
- Goodlife Health Food
- My Health Market
- Pure + Natural

Sydney
- Aboutlife
- Adora Healthy Living
- Bondi Wholefoods

- Earth Food Store
- The Farm Wholefoods
- The Health Emporium
- Macro Wholefoods Market // Woolworths
- Naked Foods
- Natural Food Market
- QVB Health Foods
- Wholefoods House

NEW ZEALAND
Auckland
- The Devonport Health Store
- The Health Store
- Little Bird Organics
- Naturally Organic
- Organic Evolution
- The Vegan Shop

Wellington
- Ceres Organics
- Commonsense Organics
- East West Organics
- Gluten Free Grocer
- The Greengrocer
- Green Trading
- Hardy's Healthy Living
- Natural Health Centre
- Take Care Health Shop and Clinic

PEOPLE'S REPUBLIC OF CHINA
Hong Kong
- Aussie Organics
- Bon Vivant Organics
- Health Essential
- Homegrown Foods
- Just Green Organic Convenience Store
- ThreeSixty Store

EUROPE

DENMARK
Copenhagen
- Øko Best
- Puregreen
- SuperBrugsen
- Torvehallerne

FRANCE
Paris
- Bio c'Bon
- Biocoop Toutelabio Paris Glacière
- Naturalia
- TouchofBio

GERMANY
Berlin
- Alnatura
- basic bio
- Bio Company
- BioInsel
- Biosphäre
- denn's Biomarkt
- Kraut & Rüben Naturkost
- LPG Biomarkt
- Naturkaufhaus
- Siebenkorn
- Veganz
- Vitalia Reformhaus
- VollCorner Biomarkt
- Wurzelwerk

Frankfurt
- Alnatura
- basic bio
- BioMarkt Picard
- tegut… gute Lebensmittel
- Veganz

Hamburg
Alnatura
Bio Company
denn's Biomarkt
Reformhaus Engelhardt
Tjaden's Bio Frischemarkt

Munich
Alnatura
basic bio
BioVolet
denn's Biomarkt
Kornkammer Naturkost
Landmann's Biomarkt
Schmatz Naturkost
Vitalia Reformhaus
VollCorner Biomarkt

ITALY
Milan
Biobene
bio.it
La bottega italiana Ca' alma
L'Elisir Erboristeria
NaturaSì

Rome
Biomens
Il Canestro
Coop Nautia
Earth Markets
La Bottega Bio

SPAIN
Madrid
Eat Organic
El Vergel
La Nodriza
Mama Campo

SWEDEN
Stockholm
8T8
Ekologiska Barnmatsbutiken
Goodstore
Gryningen
Saltå Kvarn
Smaksatt

SWITZERLAND
Geneva
Bio-Servette
Diététicontamines
L'Atelier Du Bio
Le Grain de Vie
Le Marché Bio
Marché de Vie
Marché Mini Prix
Naturdiet Sàrl (Alna)
Relais de la Nature
Votre Santé

Zurich
Biomarkthalle Vitus
Egli Plaza
Migros

UNITED KINGDOM
London
Abel & Cole
The Nutri Centre
Ocado
Planet Organic
Revital
Riverford
Whole Foods Market

MIDDLE EAST

UNITED ARAB EMIRATES
Dubai
Bio Organic Store
Blue Planet Green People
Down to Earth Organic
Health Factory
Holland & Barrett
Organic Foods and Café

NORTH AMERICA

CANADA
Montréal
A Votre Santré
Délices Bio Inc
Rachelle-Béry
Club Organic

Toronto
Vital Planet Health Shop
Essence of Life Organics
The Sweet Potato

Vancouver
Famous Foods
Greens Market
The Organic Grocer
Pomme Natural Market
Whole Foods Market

UNITED STATES OF AMERICA
Chicago
Bonne Sante Health Foods
Chicago Health Foods
Hyde Park Produce
Life Springs Health Foods & Juice Bar
Newleaf Natural Grocery
Whole Foods Market

Los Angeles
Bristol Farms
Country Natural Foods
Café Gratitude
Erewhon Market
Farmers Market
Moon Juice
Organix
Pacific Coast Greens
Sprouts Farmers Market
SunLife Organics
Trader Joe's
Whole Foods Market

Miami
Trader Joe's
Whole Foods Market

New York
Gourmet Garage
Trader Joe's
Whole Foods Market

INDEX

We believe in buying seasonal and organic produce. If you are not in a position to buy organic then we recommend making sure that your proteins such as meat, poultry, and eggs are organic and your fish is wild-caught.

CHOCOLATE
Banana Ice Cream 156
Choco Ball Bites 57
Chocolate Shortbread Cookies 143
Peanut Ball Bites 56
Vegan Chocolate Cake 138

CILANTRO
Avocado & Shrimp 92
Carrot Soup 103
Green Pea Dip 70
Guacamole Dip 74
Kimia's Falafels 82
Quinoa & Chickpea Burgers 112

CINNAMON
Almond Milk 20
Baked Doughnuts 148
Banana Oat Pancakes & Un-Nutella 34
Carrot Cupcakes 62
Cinnamon Popcorn 58
Cinnamon Tea 26
FTF Almond Butter 161
Ginger Snap Cookies 54
Granola 46
Hug in a Mug Hot Cocoa 24
Millet Granola 42
Nice Cream Cookie Sandwich 154
Peanut Ball Bites 56
Porridge 38
Summer Bircher Muesli 48
Super Seed Crackers 76

COCONUT
Carrot Cupcakes 62
Chia Breakfast Pot 40
Choco Princess Layer Slice 136
Cod Fish fingers with Coconut 91
FTF Almond Butter 161
Nice Cream Cookie Sandwich 154
Summer Bircher Muesli 48
Walnut Ball Bites 57

COCONUT CREAM
Banana Ice Cream 156
Chia Breakfast Pot 40
Nice Cream Cookie Sandwich 154

COCONUT FLOUR
Berry Cheesecake Muffins 64

COCONUT MILK
Baked Doughnuts 148
Banana Oat Pancakes & Un-Nutella 34
Choco Princess Layer Slice 136
Raw Cacao & Avocado Mousse 134
Summer Bircher Muesli 48
Vegan Chocolate Cake 138

COCONUT NECTAR
FTF Raw Berry Jam 160

COCONUT SUGAR
Baked Doughnuts 148
Cacao Beet Brownies 146
Esti & Gekko's Pumpkin Soup 96
FTF Shortbread Pastry 142
Ginger Snap Cookies 54

COCONUT WATER
FTF Raw Berry Jam 160
Mermaid Smoothie 28

COCONUT YOGURT
Baba's Froyo 66
Banana Orange Ice Lolly 60
Berry Cheesecake Muffins 64
Kimia's Falafels 82
Millet Breakfast Pot 44
Nice Cream Cookie Sandwich 154
Summer Bircher Muesli 48

COD
Cod Fish Fingers with coconut 91

CORN
Cinnamon Popcorn 58

CORN FLOUR
Green Fritters 84

COTTAGE CHEESE
Banana Oat Pancakes & Un-Nutella 34

CRANBERRIES
Granola 46
Turkey Stew 100

CREAM CHEESE
Carrot Cupcakes 62

CUCUMBER
Avocado Cucumber Roll 90
Mackerel & Sardine Pate 78

CUMIN
Esti & Gekko's Pumpkin Soup 96
Kimia's Falafels 82
Quinoa & Chickpea Burgers 112

CURRY POWDER
Esti & Gekko's Pumpkin Soup 96

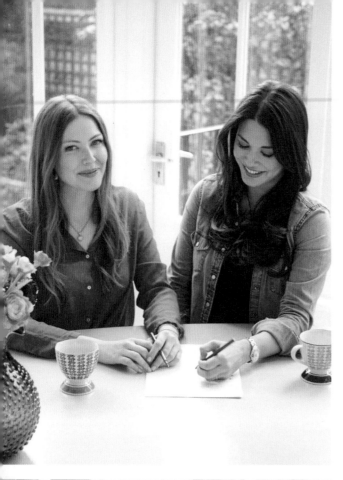
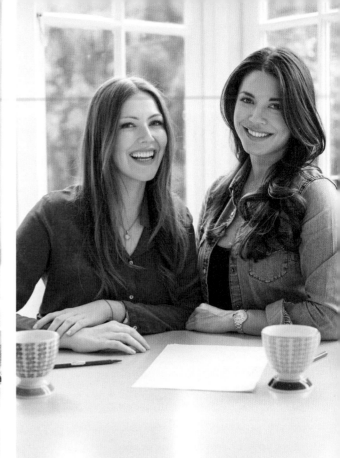
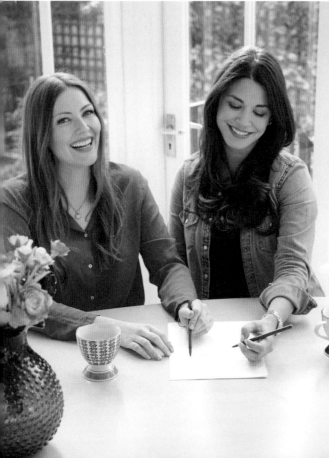
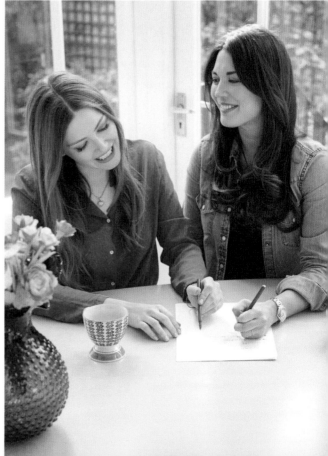

THANK YOUS

LOHRALEE

This book has been a great joy to work on every step of the way, from writing, to coming up with fun, tasty recipes, to testing all of our creations. To my dear friend, Tali, thank you for being such a joy to work with. Will, my husband, has been incredibly supportive as have my two little ones, Waldorf and Allegra. Thank you for for being our little critics by tasting and approving all the recipes! I am incredibly grateful to all of my dear family and friends that have supported me through this journey. A special thank you to Alice Sheffield, Rob Gilbert, Lisa Henrekson, Bella Musgrave, Emily Goad, Elizabeth Rafferty, and Richard Dennen.

TALI

Thank you to my beautiful and talented partner and friend, Lohralee Astor, as well as Will, Waldorf, and Allegra. Thank you also to these amazing people for their friendship, love, support, and advice throughout this project and beyond; Siobhan Kennelly, Jamie, Orla and Niamh Tomlinson, Malin, Coco and Rex Jefferies, Julia, Estelle and Felix Zaouk, Sogol Samadi, Alex Spencer-Churchill, Adriana, Raphaela and Nathanial Weiss, Caroline Marcus, Samantha Brett, Nicky and Bruce McWilliam, Angelique Andrews, Skye McDonald, Joe Farage, Lynda and Lauren Prince, Lauren Sandler, and of course my own Papa bear, Adrian Shine.

LOHRALEE & TALI

We have been incredibly lucky to have our friend Patrycia as our talented photographer. Your photographs are beautiful and have filled the book with laughter and color. Thank you for bringing this book to life. Thank you to Hendrik, Regina, Regine, and everyone else at teNeues for their dedication, input, and commitment to making this book.

A special thank you to Oka Direct for the china and flowers used during the shoot, to Sadaf Ahmad for the beautiful makeup, to Jack Merrick-Thirlway from Neville Hair & Beauty Salon for our hairstyling, and to Melanie Haizmann and Regina Denk for cooking and styling.

More thanks to www.kaufdichgruen.de, your webshop for disposable tableware and drinking cups made from renewable and recycled raw materials, sustainable food packaging, and organic products for home and garden.

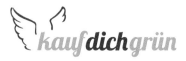

IMPRINT

© 2016 teNeues Media GmbH & Co. KG, Kempen

Texts by Tali Shine & Lohralee Astor
Photos by Patrycia Lukas

Editorial management by Regine Freyberg
Copy editing by Natalie Compton
Production by Nele Jansen
Imaging & proofing by David Burghardt/db-photo.de

Published by teNeues Publishing Group

teNeues Media GmbH + Co. KG
Am Selder 37, 47906 Kempen, Germany
Phone: +49 (0)2152 916 0
Fax: +49 (0)2152 916 111
e-mail: books@teneues.com

Press department: Andrea Rehn
Phone: +49 (0)2152 916 202
e-mail: arehn@teneues.com

teNeues Publishing Company
7 West 18th Street, New York, NY 10011, USA
Phone: +1 212 627 9090
Fax: +1 212 627 9511

teNeues Publishing UK Ltd.
12 Ferndene Road, London SE24 0AQ, UK
Phone: +44 (0)20 3542 8997

teNeues France S.A.R.L.
39, rue des Billets, 18250 Henrichemont, France
Phone: +33 (0)2 48 26 93 48
Fax: +33 (0)1 70 72 34 82

www.teneues.com

ISBN: 978-3-8327-3343-8
Library of Congress Control Number: 2015958062
Printed in Spain by Estellaprint

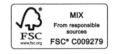